Fashionable Clothing from the Sears Catalogs

LATE *1930s*

Tammy Ward
Tina Skinner

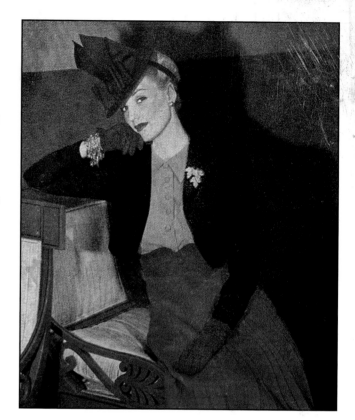

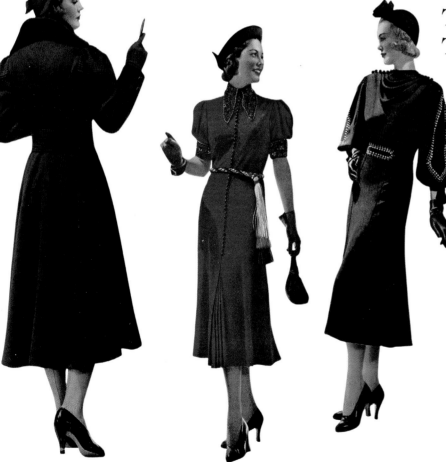

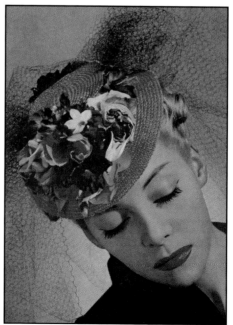

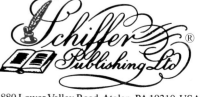
4880 Lower Valley Road, Atglen, PA 19310 USA

About the Authors

Tammy Ward is a fashion-conscious writer from Southeastern Pennsylvania.

Tina Skinner is a professional editor and writer who specializes in design.

Copyright © 2006 by Schiffer Publishing Ltd.
Library of Congress Control Number: 2006924594

All rights reserved. No part of this work may be reproduced or used in any form or by any means—graphic, electronic, or mechanical, including photocopying or information storage and retrieval systems—without written permission from the publisher.
The scanning, uploading and distribution of this book or any part thereof via the Internet or via any other means without the permission of the publisher is illegal and punishable by law. Please purchase only authorized editions and do not participate in or encourage the electronic piracy of copyrighted materials.
"Schiffer," "Schiffer Publishing Ltd. & Design," and the "Design of pen and ink well" are registered trademarks of Schiffer Publishing Ltd.

Designed by John P. Cheek
Cover design by Bruce Waters
Type set in Zurich BT

ISBN: 0-7643-2485-3
Printed in China

Published by Schiffer Publishing Ltd.
4880 Lower Valley Road
Atglen, PA 19310
Phone: (610) 593-1777
Fax: (610) 593-2002
E-mail: Info@schifferbooks.com

For the largest selection of fine reference books on this and related subjects, please visit our web site at **www.schifferbooks.com**
We are always looking for people to write books on new and related subjects. If you have an idea for a book please contact us at the above address.

This book may be purchased from the publisher.
Include $3.95 for shipping.
Please try your bookstore first.
You may write for a free catalog.

In Europe, Schiffer books are distributed by
Bushwood Books
6 Marksbury Ave.
Kew Gardens
Surrey TW9 4JF England
Phone: 44 (0) 20 8392-8585
Fax: 44 (0) 20 8392-9876
E-mail: info@bushwoodbooks.co.uk
Website: www.bushwoodbooks.co.uk
Free postage in the U.K., Europe; air mail at cost.

Dedication

To Joe Martinow, a fashion genius with remarkable market insight.

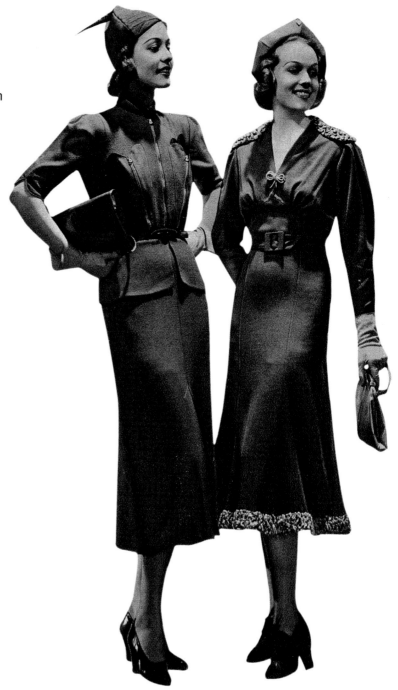

Catalog Pages Used

Fall/Winter 1936-37
6, 7, 8, 9, 11, 12, 13, 16, 20, 31, 32, 35, 46, 62, 71, 83, 85, 91, 107, 139, 146, 150, 156, 217, 306, 307, 312, 336, 340, 342, 360, 362, 365, 375, 376

Fall/Winter 1939-1940
2, 3, 4, 5, 7, 13, 17, 20, 21, 22, 25, 27, 30, 33, 36, 39, 43, 47, 51, 53, 55, 59, 60, 69, 71, 78, 80, 81, 88, 89, 92, 96, 109, 203, 204, 205, 206, 219, 221, 238, 250, 257, 258, 289, 332, 334, 337, 344, 345, 347, 348, 350, 364, 380, 402, 404A, 404C, 405, 408, 420A, 420B, 421, 422, 424, 425, 435, 462, 463, 464, 465, 466, 467, 469, 470A, 470D, 471, 475, 479, 497, 499, 501

Spring/Summer 1939
2, 10, 13, 16, 18, 24, 25, 33, 38, 48, 53, 64, 67, 84, 90, 93, 163, 165, 193, 226, 228, 254, 256, 259, 282, 290, 295, 341, 351, 353

Spring/Summer 1937
1, 6, 7, 8, 9, 11, 12, 14, 16, 29, 33, 37, 52, 53, 73, 74, 77, 81, 84, 85, 89, 92, 93, 155, 157, 161, 173, 267, 268, 279, 281, 284, 286, 287, 288, 289, 294

Spring/Summer 1938
2, 4, 11, 13, 16, 19, 24, 26, 28, 33, 35, 36, 38, 45, 55, 58, 61, 70, 73, 76, 78, 80, 83, 84, 104, 123, 141, 143, 172, 181, 183, 184, 213, 215, 234, 244, 245, 306

Fall/Winter 1938-1939
4, 7, 15, 21, 23, 25, 26, 32, 34, 36, 37, 38, 43, 44, 49, 51, 52, 54, 57, 62, 63, 67, 69, 75, 81, 83, 87, 125, 149, 151, 157, 158, 169, 171, 174, 175, 219, 221, 223, 225, 231, 234, 280, 302, 305, 306, 307, 311, 315, 317, 337, 340, 341, 355, 369, 376, 377, 420, 422, 423, 429, 439

Fall/Winter 1937-38
IFC, 1, 2, 3, 4, 5, 6, 7, 8, 11, 13, 15, 18, 24, 26, 29, 36, 37, 38, 39, 40, 45, 48, 54, 60, 65, 67, 71, 86, 87, 93, 95, 96, 97, 100, 105, 108, 110, 115, 117, 124, 126, 127, 131, 133, 134, 135, 138, 142, 148, 156, 159, 161, 172, 177, 202, 203, 205, 215, 221, 223, 243, 245, 248, 252, 254, 255, 279, 282, 292, 296, 298, 299, 306, 308, 314, 315, 316, 324, 326, 327, 329, 330, 333, 334, 355, 359, 367, 368, 371, 385, 389, 402, 405, 416, 418, 427, 428, 429

Contents

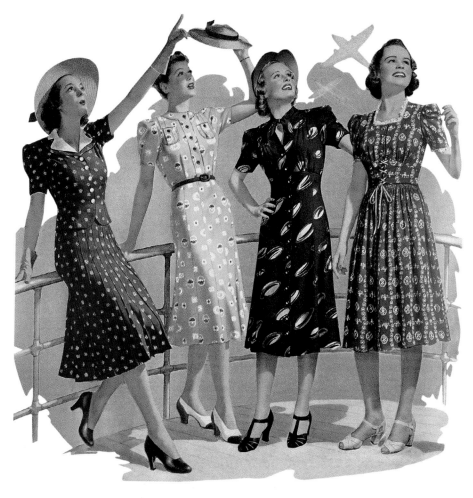

Introduction

The 1930s was an era gripped by The Great Depression. Money was scarce, the average income was $1,400 annually, unemployment was prevalent, and the Great American dream started to become a nightmare for many, so Americans did what they could to make life a happier time. Movies including *Snow White & The Seven Dwarfs*, *Scarface*, *The Mummy*, *King Kong*, and the introduction of America's Sweetheart, Shirley Temple, all helped to entertain America. Board games (such as the still popular game Monopoly), Nancy Drew mysteries, radio programs such as Amos 'n Andy, Little Orphan Annie, The Lone Ranger, Buck Rogers, and dancing to the sounds of the big bands were all a source of escape to help ease the burden of living in these desperate times.

Franklin Delano Roosevelt was president of the United States through much of the 1930s, while great changes took place on the political, social, and science fronts of this era. A small sample of some of these important events include: *The Star Spangled Banner* became the national anthem in America, Adolf Hitler became chancellor in Germany, Alcatraz Maximum Security Prison opened, Amelia Earhart was the first person to attempt to fly solo across the Pacific Ocean, the lie detector machine was invented, the Home Owners Loan Act was endorsed to boost home building, the first claims for Social Security were paid, General Motors mass produced the diesel engine, and the New York World's Fair was aired for the first time on television.

The Autumn, 1930 Sears Catalogue admonished, "Thrift is the spirit of the day. Reckless spending is a thing of the past." American designers came into their own during this era since fashions from Paris were now unaffordable to all but the very rich. Hollywood stars such as Gretta Garbo and Bette Davis helped to set the fashion trends of this era. Zippers replaced the more expensive button, hem lines changed with the hour of the day, mid calf for day, long for evening. A more feminine look evolved, replacing the boyish look of the '20s. The waist of the dresses and skirts returned to the natural waistline and necklines dropped and were often accentuated with inset pieces and yolks. Skirts were full and had lots of gathers or layers. Trains were added to gowns to add a formal touch. Fur of any type was very popular for day or evening wear. Hats were often worn at an angle and pill boxes became stylish.

This era brought to fruition the "Age of Comfort." Gone was the stiff shirt collar and formality in men's wear of previous times. For men, pants were worn high on the waist with a wide waistband, vest sweaters replaced the matching vest of a three-piece suit, blazers and linen pants were worn together. Double-breasted suits such as the Windsor and the Kent were popular. These were made fashionable by such actors as Clark Gable, Cary Grant, and Fred Astaire, who endorsed these suits by wearing them in their movies. Also popular was the famous "Palm Beach" suit. It was considered the Wall Street businessman's suit. Gangsters projected the image of businessmen by wearing suits, easily recognizable by the bolder, wider stripes, pronounced shoulders, narrower waists, and more colorful ties. Whether actors, businessmen, or gangsters, no well-dressed man was complete without a stylish hat to top it all off.

Homemakers of the 1930s would mend and patch clothing before replacing it. Fabrics that were washable, lightweight, and easy to care for were introduced in this era of the thrifty shopper. Cheaper fabrics were used to make clothing. Cotton was no longer considered a cheap fabric used just for work clothes. Designers began to work enthusiastically with rayon as it dyed well and gave the appearance of silk to women's lingerie.

The 1930s were not just gloom and doom. For many it was very hard just to survive, but there were good and positive changes for many as well. To name a few, it became the age of physical fitness, and getting more exercise became an important factor to the well being of men, women, and children. Women started wearing trousers and earned more personal freedoms such as working outside of the home to help pay the bills. Discrimination toward people of color was beginning to change as Eleanor Roosevelt became an active champion of black rights, and this was considered to be a major step forward for the rights of black Americans.

Pictured in this book are fashion images of men, women, and children taken from the Sears catalogs throughout the 1930s. These images give us a look at what people were wearing in the business world, casual day to day living, and evening wear. Historians, collectors, and designers will be fascinated by the images of an era gone by.

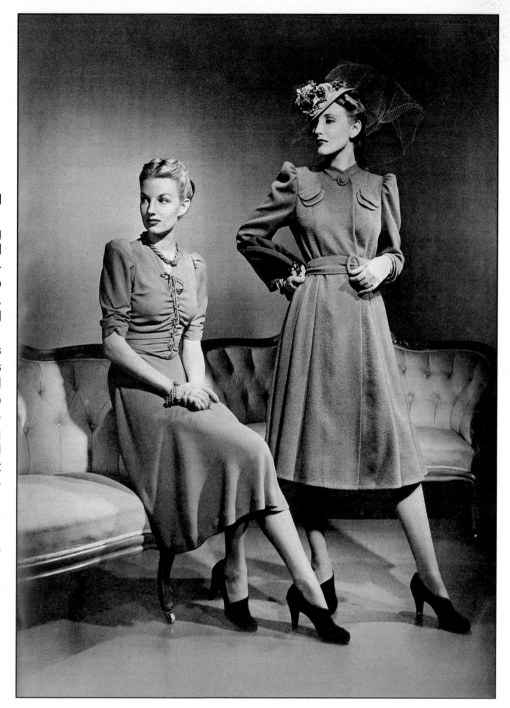

Women's Fashions

Gowns

Enchanting evening gown has a dramatic off-the-shoulder neckline, a boned bodice that accentuates a tiny waist, a full seven yards of billowing ruffles on a flaring skirt. Wear it with or without the shoulder straps and removable hoop. A rustling Rayon Taffeta petticoat is attached to the dress. Made of lustrous Rayon Net, a filmy, fragile-looking fabric, it is the perfect choice for this romantic fashion. This beautiful gown comes in Romance Aqua, Petal Pink, or White. *Spring/Summer 1939*

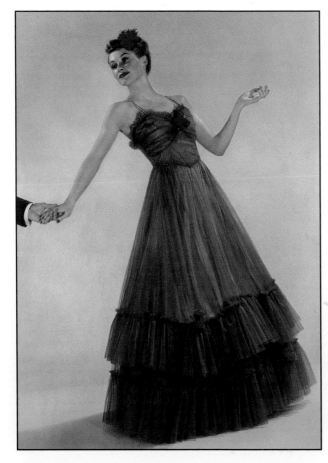

Daguerreotype dress of Rayon Taffeta embossed with old-fashioned flowers. High in back and cuts to a moderately low square in the front. Butterfly wings sleeves and whirligig skirt. Bouffant dress with Bolero Jacket is Celanese Rayon Taffeta with rayon velvet ribbons. Hoop style skirt with low-backed frock. Celanese Rayon Panné Satin dinner gown has contrasting gardenias nestled at the neckline and trim the flaring draped hemline. *Fall/Winter 1939-1940*

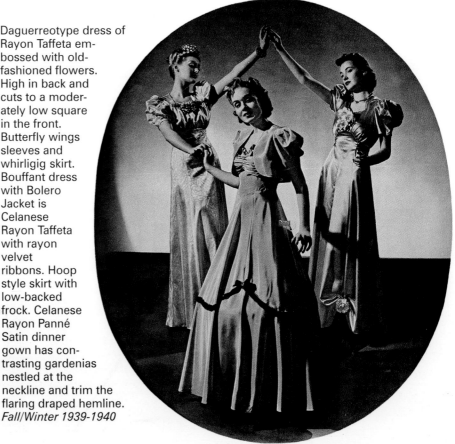

Romantic junior gowns in "Evening Star", "Prom Trotter", and "Shining Hour" styles. "Snow Bunny" wrap will compliment any of these glamorous gowns. *Fall/Winter 1938/1939*

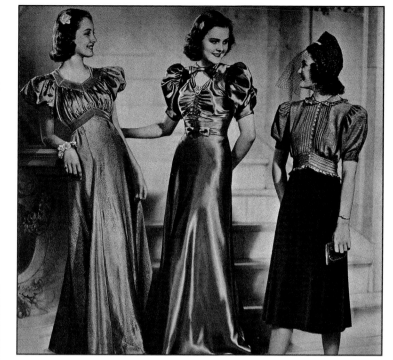

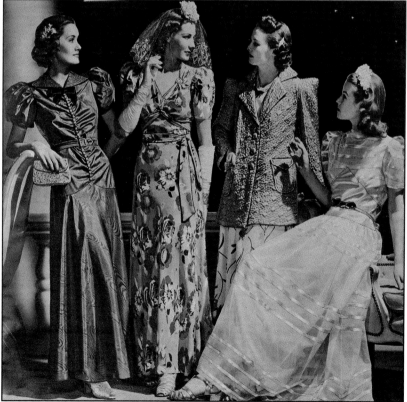

Moire Rayon Taffeta party dress with puffed short sleeves, pointed revers have rows of fine stitching, and self-covered buttons from neck to hip. Floral pattern Tiara French-Type Rayon Crepe has the new form-revealing line that slims the waist and rounds up the bosom. Quilted Rayon Taffeta short evening coat is the backbone of every girl's wardrobe with square, boxed shoulders, and soft enough not to crush your daintiest frocks. Yards and yards of Rayon Marquisette sheer striped satin are used in the skirt and top of this gown, it has a wide V-shaped Rayon Satin "girdle" about the middle, and color slip of Rayon Taffeta. *Spring/Summer 1938*

Lovely dress for a bride or bridesmaid. Made of Panne Satin of Celanese with puff sleeves, flaring corded peplum, full swirling skirt, and beautiful satin flowers. In White, Light Blue, Pink, or Maize. Movie star style is captured in "Glamour Girls" and "Hollywood Nights" dancing gowns, their designs come straight from Hollywood. Exquisite lace gown with rippling flared peplum and full shirred sleeves, and a grosgrain tieback belt. *Spring/Summer 1937*

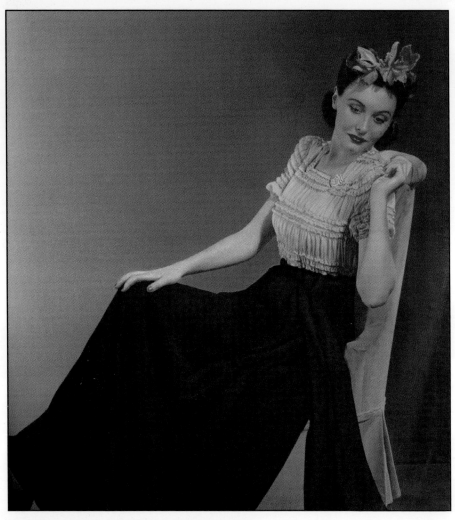

Formal length rayon pebble crepe skirt is 43" long paired with a sheer rayon chiffon blouse. This combination is the pet of Paris, the darling of New York-new, pretty, becoming. *Fall/Winter 1939-1940*

Enchanting and glamorous gowns to dance, dance, dance in! Glorious satin woven of genuine Celanese yarn, bias cut, and Nevagape adjustable placket. All rayon Moire Taffeta has fine shirring, a sash tied in back, and Nevagape placket. Beautifully patterned all rayon lace with matching slip of rayon taffeta, caplet edged with pleated net, cowled in back, and Nevagape placket. *Fall/Winter 1937-1938*

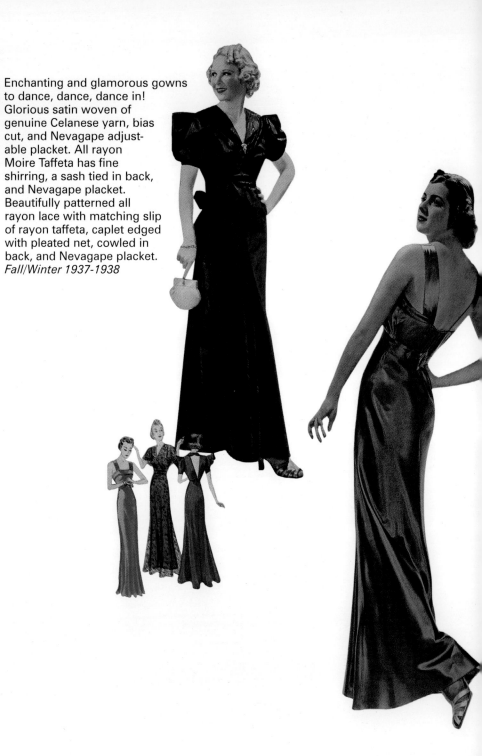

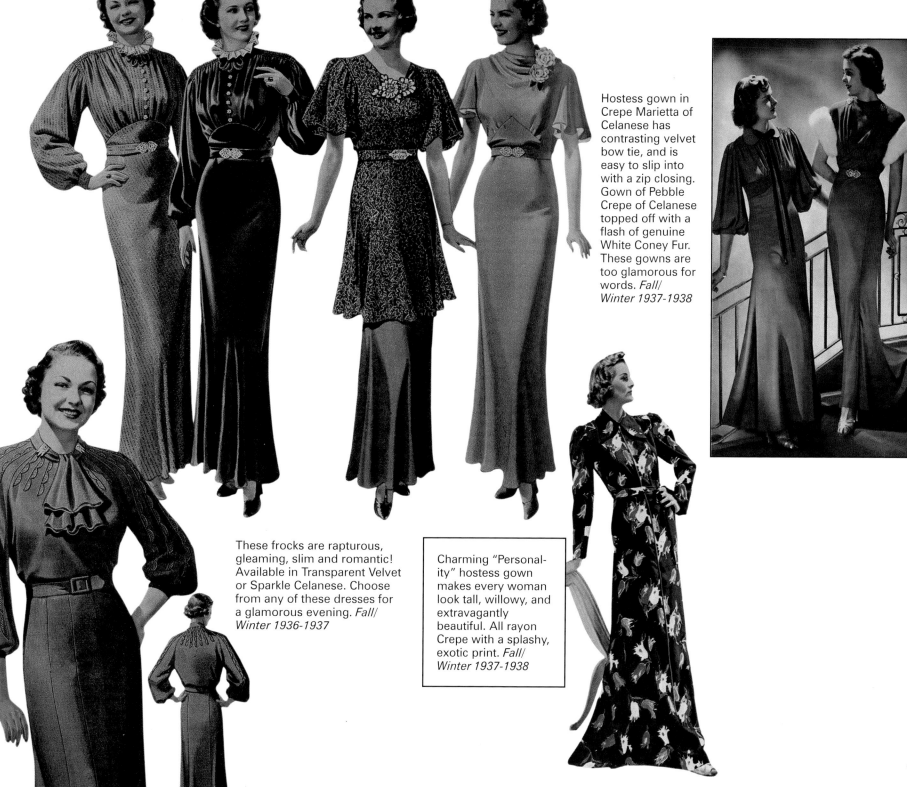

Hostess gown in Crepe Marietta of Celanese has contrasting velvet bow tie, and is easy to slip into with a zip closing. Gown of Pebble Crepe of Celanese topped off with a flash of genuine White Coney Fur. These gowns are too glamorous for words. *Fall/Winter 1937-1938*

These frocks are rapturous, gleaming, slim and romantic! Available in Transparent Velvet or Sparkle Celanese. Choose from any of these dresses for a glamorous evening. *Fall/Winter 1936-1937*

Charming "Personality" hostess gown makes every woman look tall, willowy, and extravagantly beautiful. All rayon Crepe with a splashy, exotic print. *Fall/Winter 1937-1938*

11

Career

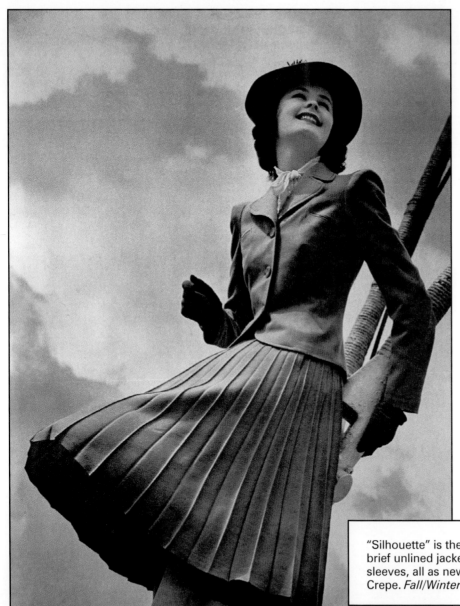

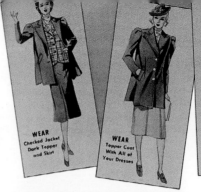

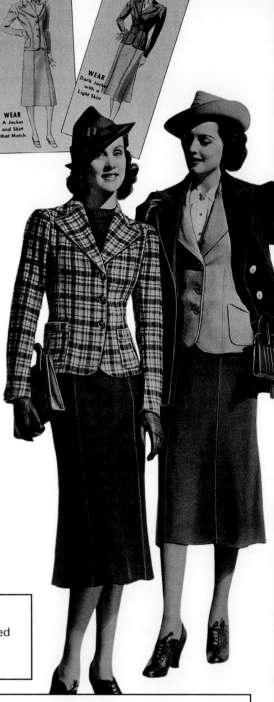

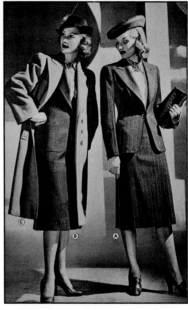

Man-Tailored suit with boxy Swagger Topcoat, both flawlessly tailored, with padded shoulders. Striped Man-Tailored suit in All Wool with a close, firm, even weave. All are ultra-smart! *Spring/Summer 1939*

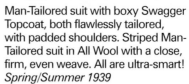

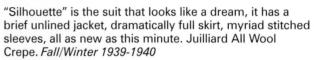

"Silhouette" is the suit that looks like a dream, it has a brief unlined jacket, dramatically full skirt, myriad stitched sleeves, all as new as this minute. Juilliard All Wool Crepe. *Fall/Winter 1939-1940*

Shetland Tweed jackets, topcoats, and skirts in matching or contrasting colors to mix and match as you please. *Spring/Summer 1938*

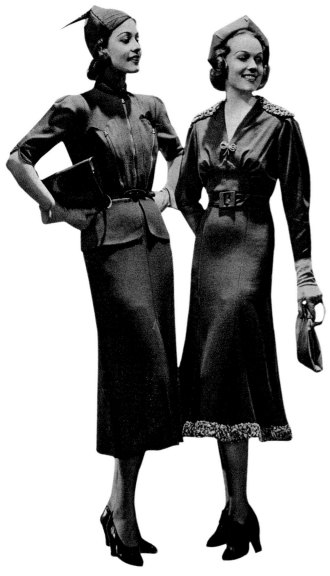

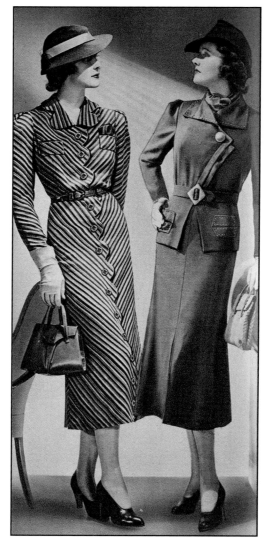

Striped spun rayon challis dress with a scalloped collar is so eye catching with its stripes and scallops. 2-piece dress with saddle stitching is all the rage in Frosty Heather spun rayon and wool. *Fall/Winter 1937-1938*

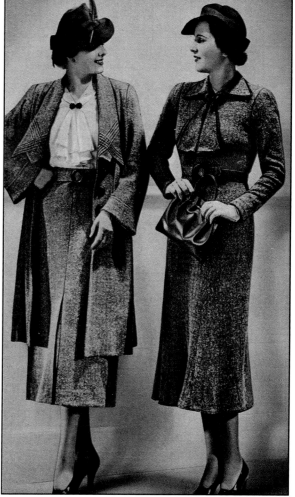

Frosty Heather-spun 2-piece dress has ascot scarf, kerchief and piping of Pebble Crepe match the zips in color. Gray Astrakhan Fur fabric accents Heather spun Princess frock, has softly draped bodice, full swing skirt, and attractive pin. Suit dress of spun rayon and wool flannel, jacket has wide shoulders, Ascot scarf, and leather effect belt in contrasting color. Hat is felt with jaunty rolled brim with wide grosgrain band. *Fall/Winter 1937-1938*

Fine tailored coat and dress of knitted tweed, blouse is of Celanese Crepe with short sleeves, jabot, and novelty pin. Knitted wool and cotton tweed is wrinkle resistant, collar and jabot are edged with contrasting Velveteen, with velveteen frog closing. *Fall/Winter 1937-1938*

Uniforms

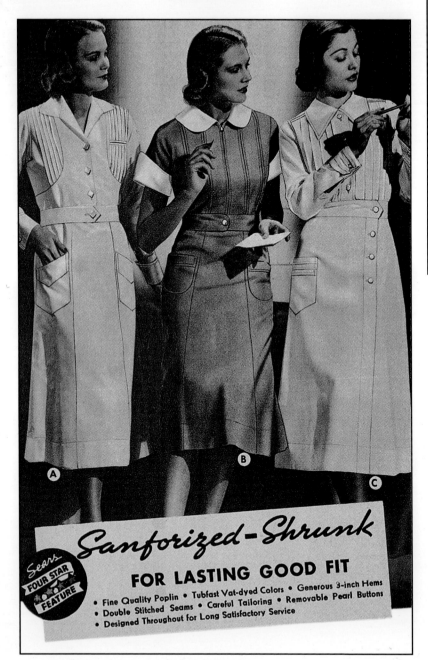

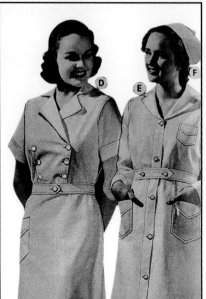

Uniforms in a variety of styles including, button-up or zip-up fronts, wrap around, or slip on, for professionals or housewives. *Spring/Summer 1938*

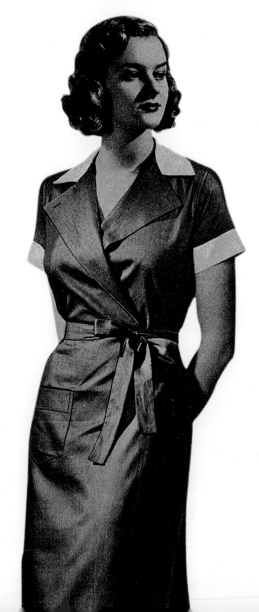

Sanforized-Shrunk

FOR LASTING GOOD FIT

- Fine Quality Poplin • Tubfast Vat-dyed Colors • Generous 3-inch Hems
- Double Stitched Seams • Careful Tailoring • Removable Pearl Buttons
- Designed Throughout for Long Satisfactory Service

Sears FOUR STAR FEATURE

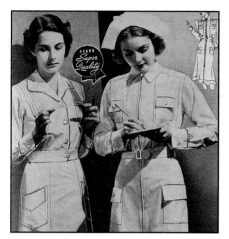

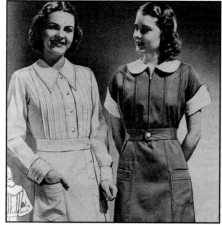

For the modern working woman, Sears has a wide variety of professional uniforms that will fit you and your job. *Fall/Winter 1938/1939*

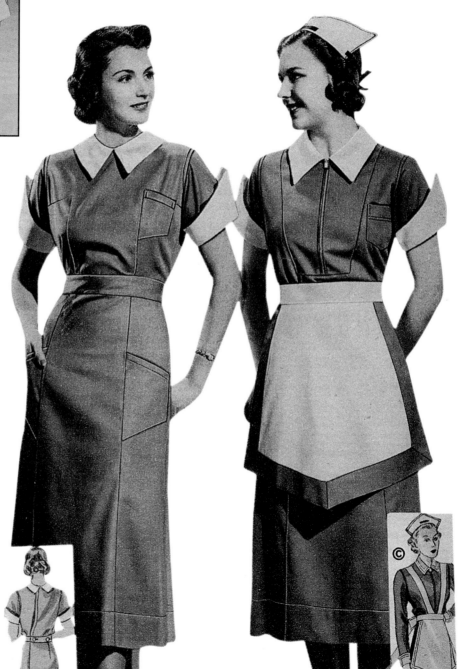

Dressy Dresses

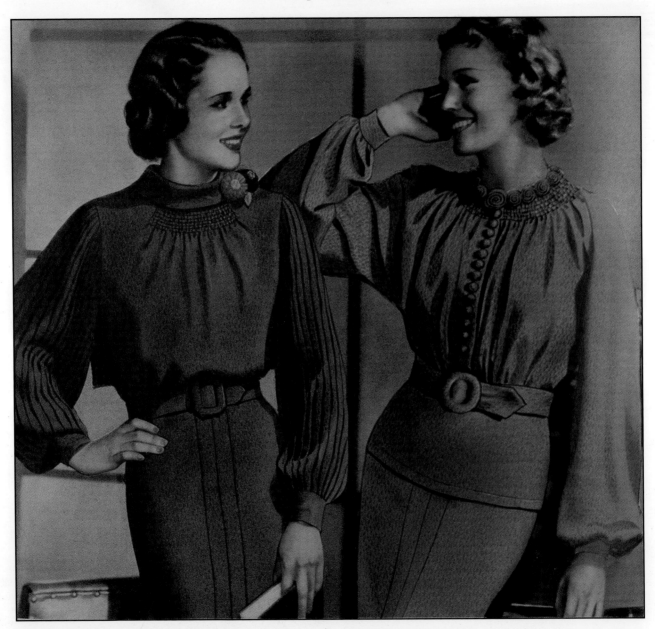

Dresses of Marietta Crepe with gorgeous big sleeves, cascades of fluttering graceful pleats, *hand made* scroll-work neckline, two-piece effect, and wide hem lines all create a luxurious effect and feel. *Fall/Winter 1936-1937*

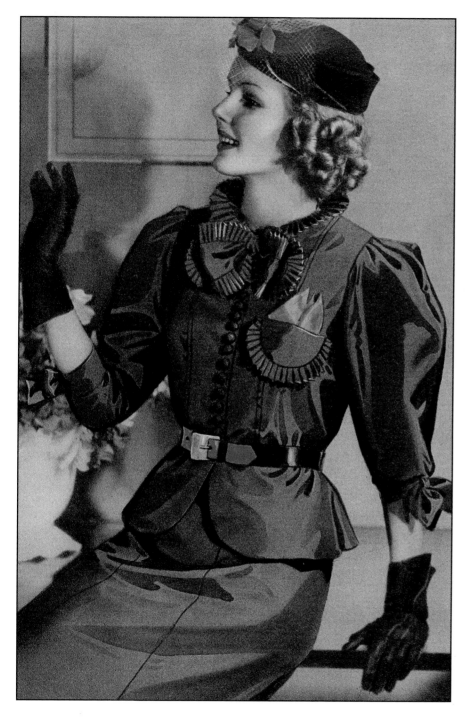

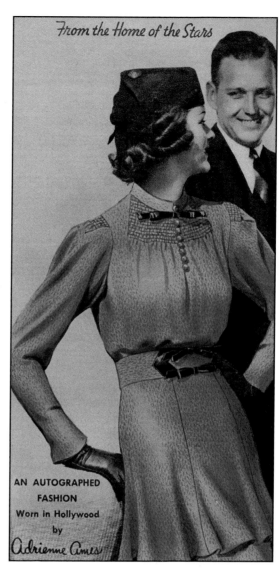

Worn in Hollywood by Adrienne Ames, and called the "lampshade tunic dress" because it flares so perkily away from the slim gored underskirt. In Marietta Crepe, it has a swank high neckline, buttons, loads of shirring, and shining patent bows at throat and belt. *Fall/Winter 1936-1937*

Taffeta or Pebble Crepe in genuine Celanese with flared peplum, a pert bow, puffy sleeves that tie with a flirty bow, a gay hankie, belt, and pleats along the bottom creating a petticoat effect all come together to make an exquisitely beautiful dress. *Fall/Winter 1936-1937*

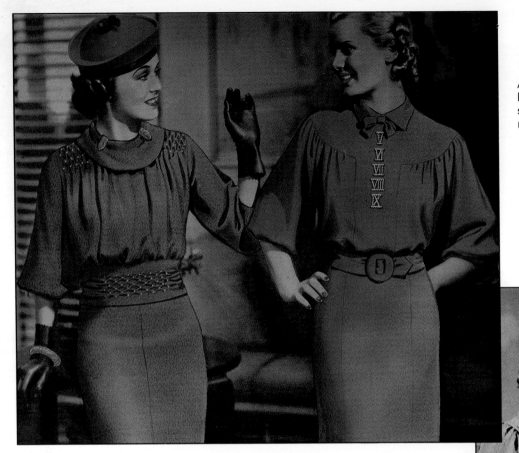

A hand smocked dress and the "Date Frock", both of Celanese, gives a feeling of "expensive". Add matching accessories and your ready for work or play. *Fall/Winter 1936-1937*

Richly textured dresses made of Celanese Matelassé gives these dresses a look of glamour. In Rust, Rose Wine, Royal Blue, Navy Blue, Dk. Green, and Brown. *Fall/Winter 1936-1937*

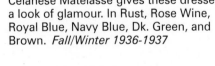

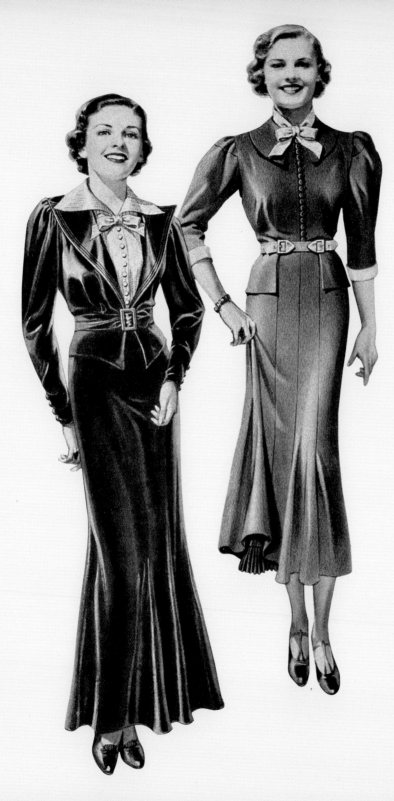

Long velvet dress, rayon faced, silk-back, and pointed down collar in Black or Royal Blue. Peplum dress in Friendship Crepe has a rustling Taffeta petticoat and detachable collar and cuffs in white Rayon Faille. Navy Blue, Spruce Green or Black. *Fall/Winter 1936-1937*

Worn in Hollywood by Anne Sothern, this satin back Crepe Amigo of Celanese dress has exquisite hand-made scroll trim, stunning pin, bracelet, and buckle that match. Soft shirring at the neck and a flared skirt combine luxuriously. Spice Brown, French Wine, and Spruce Green. *Fall/Winter 1936-1937*

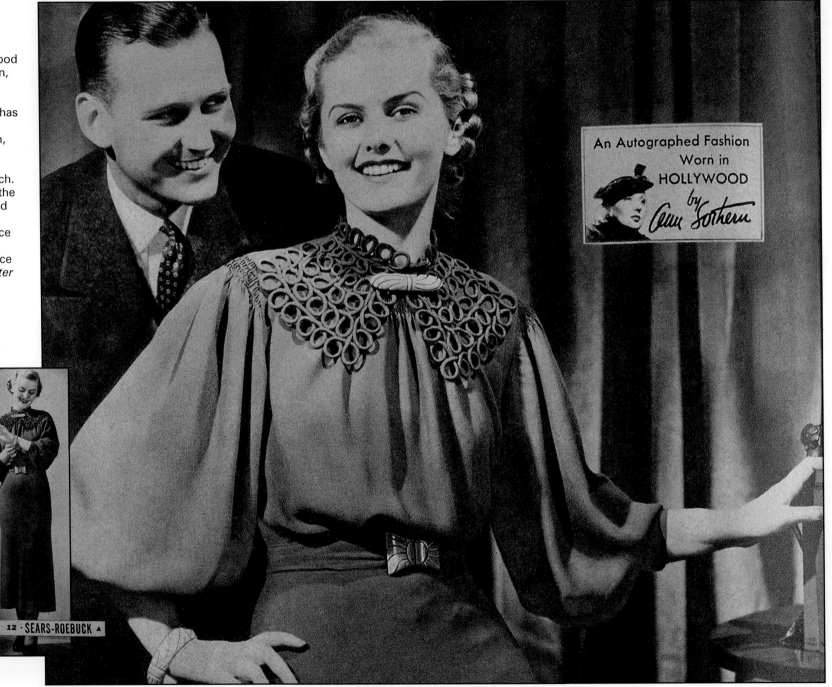

An Autographed Fashion Worn in HOLLYWOOD by *Ann Sothern*

12 · SEARS-ROEBUCK ▲

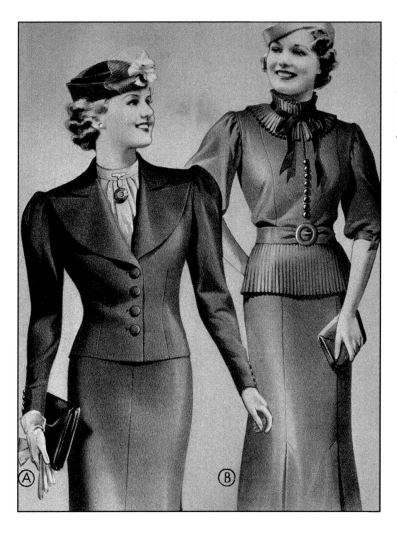

Two-piece dresses of Celanese is the fashion trend. Navy Blue with Lilac, Seal Brown, French Wine, or Rust. *Fall/Winter 1936-1937*

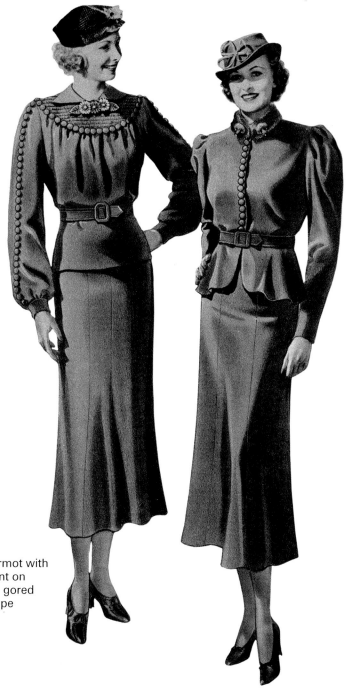

Buttons galore and fur-trimmed Mink-dyed Marmot with "Gibson Girl" sleeves makes a fashion statement on these dresses. They both have a 2-piece effect, gored skirts with a flaring hem, made with Pebble Crepe Celanese. *Fall/Winter 1936-1937*

Right:
This dress comes with a lot of variety with the option of 4 different necklines. Go from schoolgirl to glamorous with the "always right" double strand of pearls. Made of heavy Marietta Crepe of Celanese in Spruce Green, Navy Blue, or Black. *Fall/Winter 1936-1937*

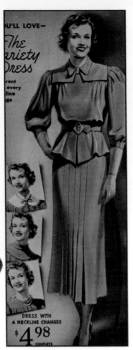

YOU'LL LOVE—
The Variety Dress

DRESS WITH
4 NECKLINE CHANGES
$4.98
COMPLETE

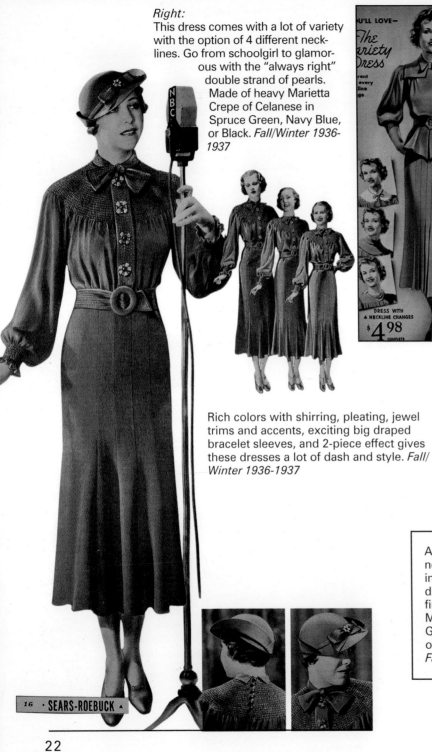

Rich colors with shirring, pleating, jewel trims and accents, exciting big draped bracelet sleeves, and 2-piece effect gives these dresses a lot of dash and style. *Fall/Winter 1936-1937*

Anne Williams has this to say about her new dress: "As I say hello, good friends, I invite you to see my new all-flattering dress. Every type, every size, every age will find it becomingly wearable!" Made of Marietta Crepe in Spice Brown, Spruce Green, French Wine, Amethyst, Navy Blue, or Rust. A matching hat is also available. *Fall/Winter 1936-1937*

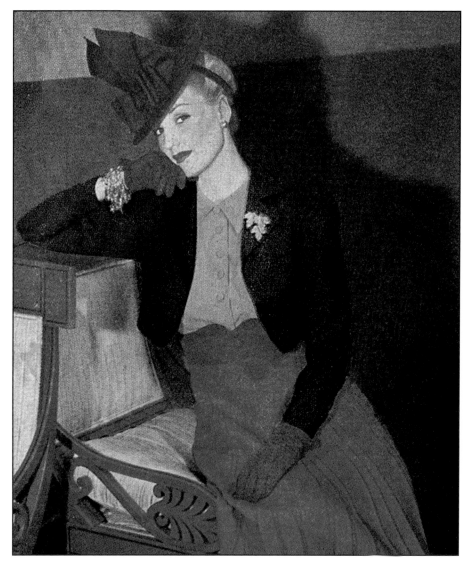

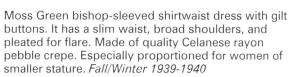

Moss Green bishop-sleeved shirtwaist dress with gilt buttons. It has a slim waist, broad shoulders, and pleated for flare. Made of quality Celanese rayon pebble crepe. Especially proportioned for women of smaller stature. *Fall/Winter 1939-1940*

A dress set that can be worn together, or individually. The skirt has permanent pleats in clusters from the hips, bolero has gold color autumn leaves on the lapel, and blouse is of Celanese Rayon Crepe Romaine. *Fall/Winter 1939-1940*

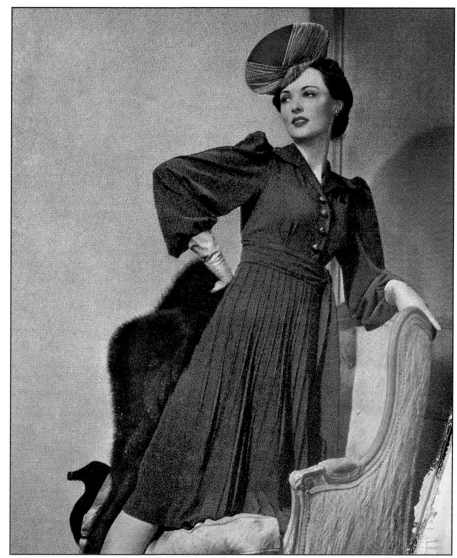

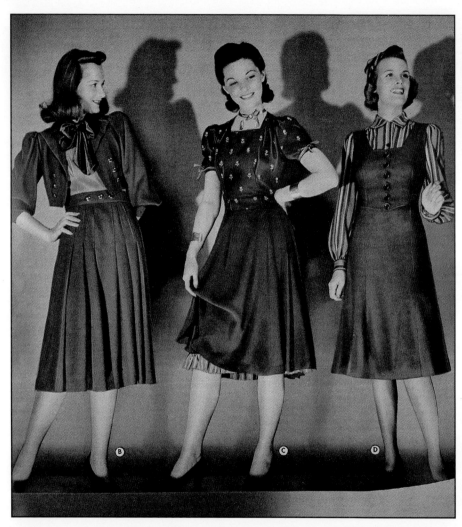

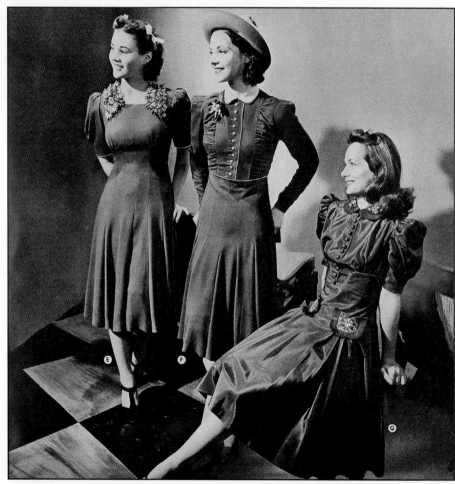

Young women love these popular dresses. The Dutch Girl dress follows the fashion trends in Holland, The Basque Girl dress has a taffeta petticoat that whispers as you walk, and The Jumper Girl dress allows for variety by wearing it with different blouses. *Fall/Winter 1939-1940*

Princess dress in Rayon Crepe is sweet simplicity with belittling effect to waist and hips, Rayon Crepe Jacket dress has flocks of buttons and is the newest fashion rage, and Celanese Rayon Taffeta dress has a tremendously full whirligig skirt that is perfect for dancing. *Fall/Winter 1939-1940*

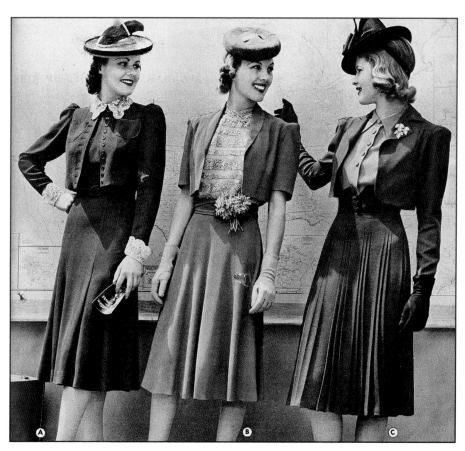

These Jacket Dresses are so pretty, so practical! They are perfect for important occasions, business, travel, and day-in day-out wear. *Fall/Winter 1939-1940*

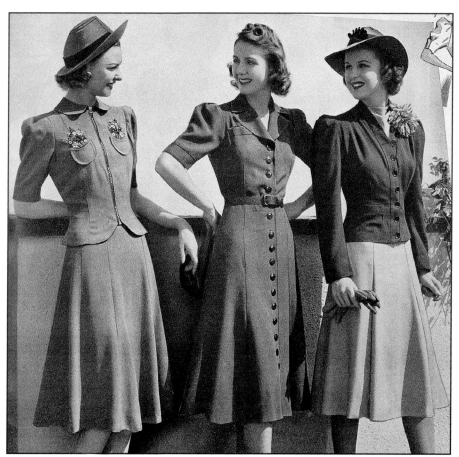

Dresses, skirts, and jackets in the newest fabric...Crown Tested Duo-Spun is spun rayon that simulates soft sheer wool. *Fall/Winter 1939-1940*

Checked top has a double-breasted effect, skirt has unpressed pleats. Bolero-effect dress is one-piece and looks expensive. Striped dress has detachable schoolgirl collar, front tucks and full skirt. And a dress that holds up to five letters to spell your name, your initials, or whatever you want! The skirt is pleated, bishop style sleeves, and "little girl" collar. *Fall/Winter 1939-1940*

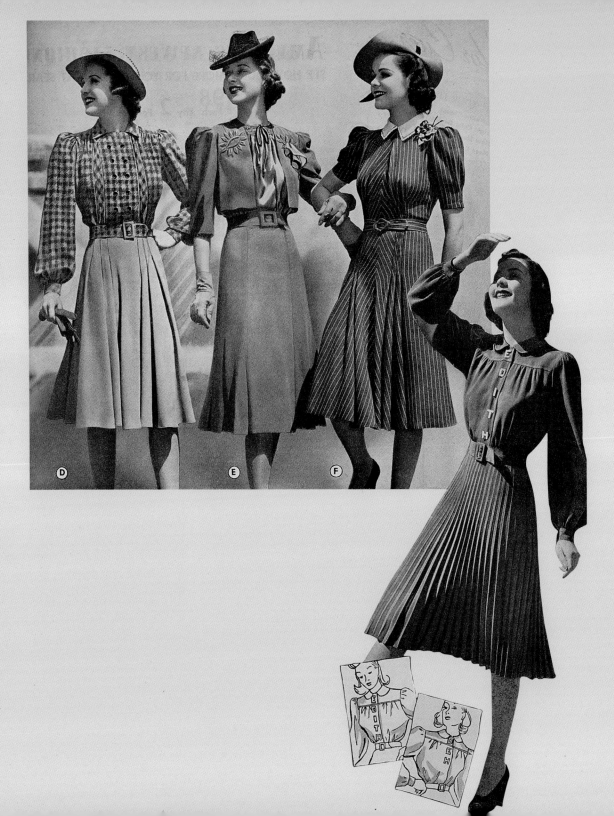

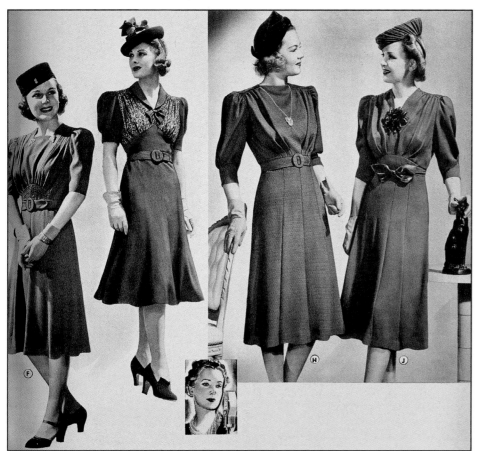

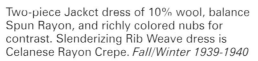

Two-piece Jacket dress of 10% wool, balance Spun Rayon, and richly colored nubs for contrast. Slenderizing Rib Weave dress is Celanese Rayon Crepe. *Fall/Winter 1939-1940*

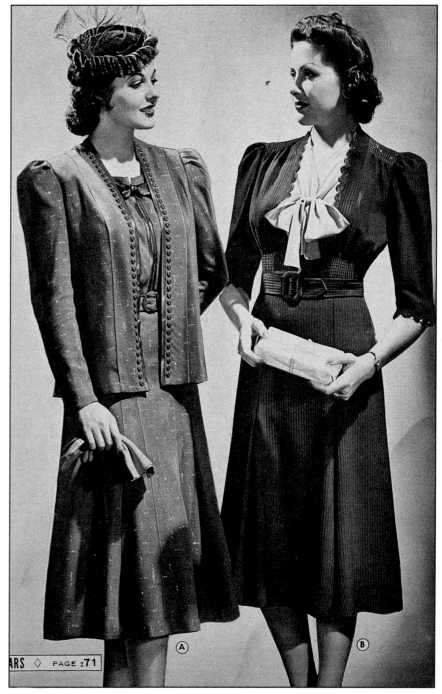

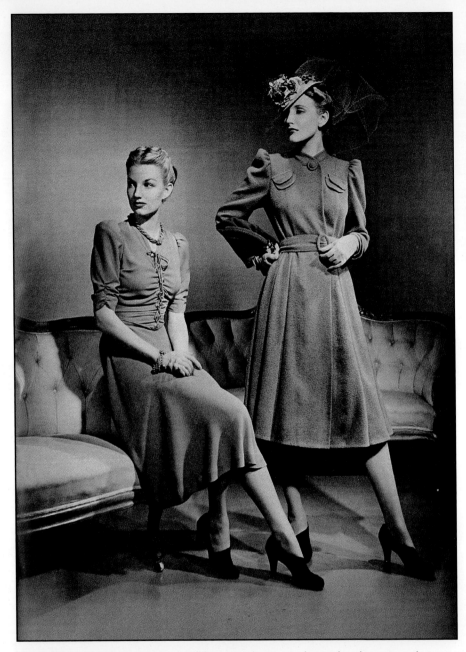

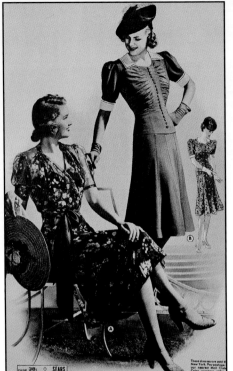

Glowing flower print dress with flattering heart-shaped neck is softly tie-draped, new gored skirt flares gracefully from the waist and has a Rayon Taffeta sash, in Silk Chiffon with Rayon Taffeta slip or in our best fabric, Rayon Berbert without the slip. Inspired from Paris, this two-piece dress has soft shirring, with draping and frosty organdy collar and cuffs. Comes in two fabrics, Celanese Rayon Crepe Romaine or Printed Rayon Crepe. *Spring/Summer 1939*

The height of fashion, these new silhouette dress are dramatic, elegant, and romantic. The daytime dress is made of soft Celanese Rayon Crepe Romaine and is cut to fit sleekly over your hips and flare wide at the hem. The Romantic Coat is modern as can be with a very new cardigan neckline and high modern pockets. It is made of All Wool Juilliard Boucle. The clever French designer, Schiaparelli, inspired its design. *Spring/Summer 1939*

Jacket and dress in Celanese Rayon Crepe Romaine has tucked shoulders, shirred bodice, and flared gored skirt. Bomberg Rayon Sheer dress is softly molded, has shirred puff sleeves, a V-neckline, and Rayon taffeta sash. Background dress of Celanese Rayon Crepe Romaine comes with bright Rhinestone clips, new below the elbow sleeves, a tucked waistline, and center pleats. *Spring/Summer 1939*

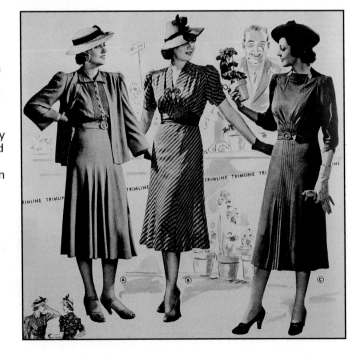

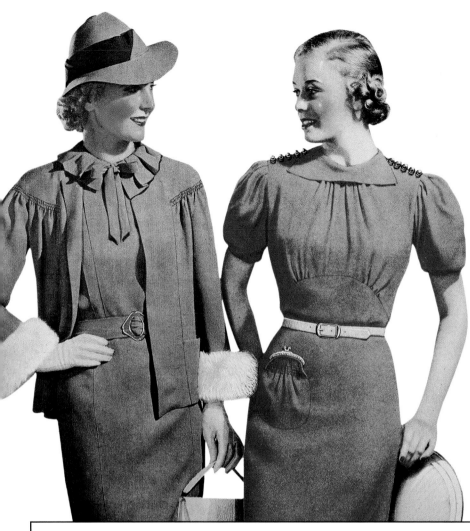

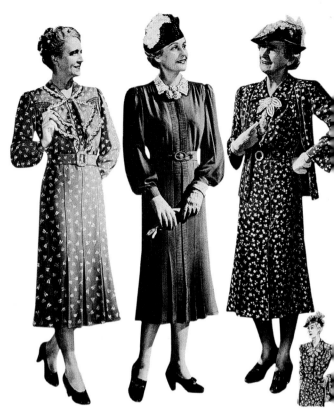

These dresses are designed to flatter our gracious ladies who are young in spirit, with softly young necklines and flared skirts. Wonderfully becoming. *Spring/Summer 1939*

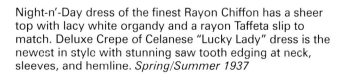

Dress and jacket of deluxe Crepe of Celanese has fluffy white fur cuffs on the jacket, pleated bodice and collar with short pleated sleeves, Pebble Crepe of Celanese dress has novelty shoulder buttons and adorable purse effect pocket. *Spring/Summer 1937*

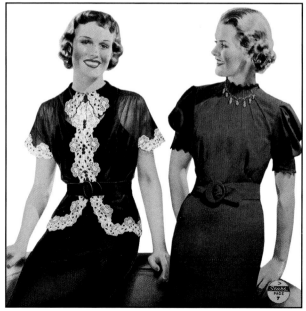

Night-n'-Day dress of the finest Rayon Chiffon has a sheer top with lacy white organdy and a rayon Taffeta slip to match. Deluxe Crepe of Celanese "Lucky Lady" dress is the newest in style with stunning saw tooth edging at neck, sleeves, and hemline. *Spring/Summer 1937*

29

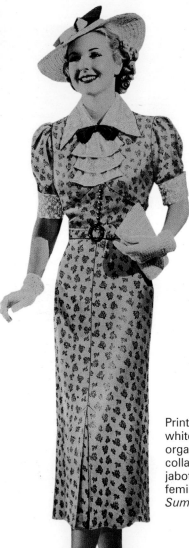

Tuxedo jacket with tuxedo revers of beautiful matching embroidery, dress has tucked front, high-tied neckline, contrast ball buttons, and a flared skirt made in Pebble Crepe of Celanese. Front dress has a hand smocked draped bustling, matching polka-dot sash and "open air" tie hat, made of Pebble Crepe of Celanese and French Finish Rayon Crepe. *Spring/Summer 1937*

Printed dress with sheer white embroidered organdy in a wide young collar with frilly three-tier jabot is so smartly feminine. *Spring/ Summer 1937*

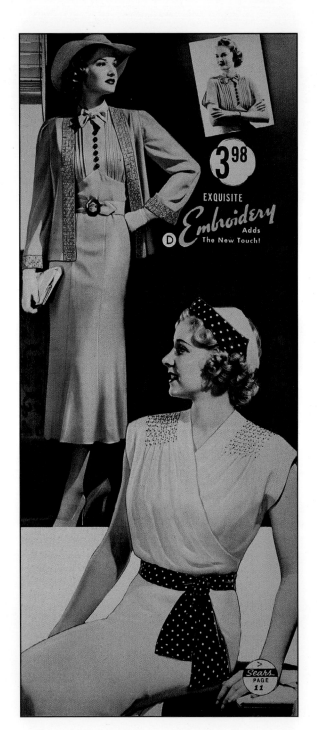

3⁹⁸

EXQUISITE Embroidery Adds The New Touch!

D

Sears PAGE 11

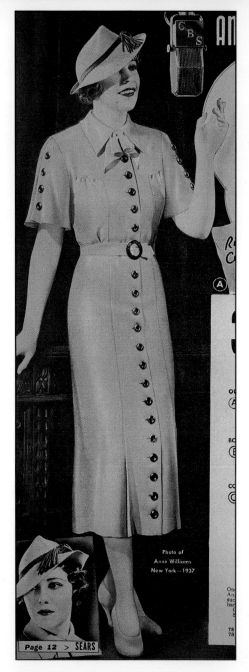

A

Photo of Anne Williams New York—1937

Page 12 > SEARS

Radio stylist Anne Williams designs this dress made of the finest DeLuxe Crepe. Buttons from neck to hem, back has an action pleat. Hat comes in either felt or straw with trim in suede leather. *Spring/ Summer 1937*

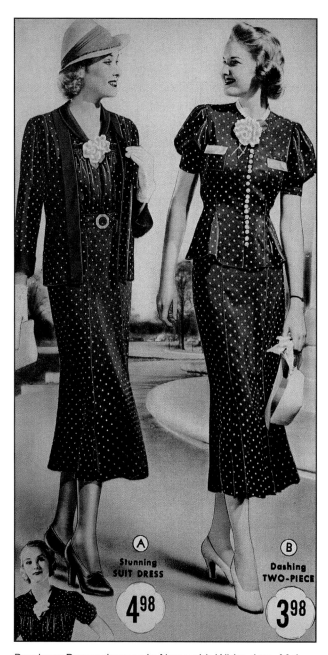

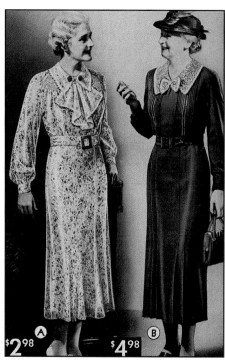

Sheer Chiffon Cotton Voile dress in a charming print has lace edged collar and jabot, soft shirring, and skirt flares in front and back. Dress of DeLuxe Crepe, it has white lace on the collar and bow, tiny tucks and rows of smart fagotting, the skirt flares in front and back. *Spring/Summer 1937*

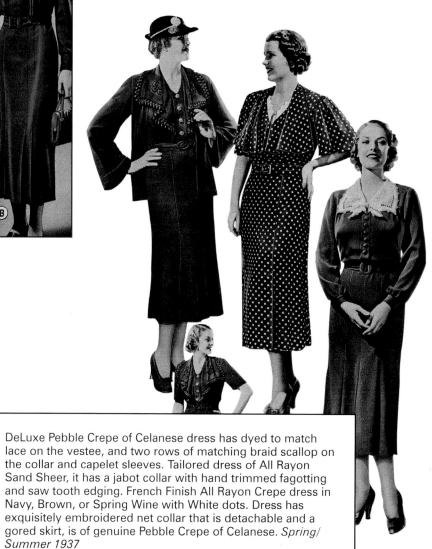

Bemberg Rayon dresses in Navy with White dots, Maize with Brown dots, or Aqua Blue with Brown dots. *Spring/ Summer 1937*

DeLuxe Pebble Crepe of Celanese dress has dyed to match lace on the vestee, and two rows of matching braid scallop on the collar and capelet sleeves. Tailored dress of All Rayon Sand Sheer, it has a jabot collar with hand trimmed fagotting and saw tooth edging. French Finish All Rayon Crepe dress in Navy, Brown, or Spring Wine with White dots. Dress has exquisitely embroidered net collar that is detachable and a gored skirt, is of genuine Pebble Crepe of Celanese. *Spring/ Summer 1937*

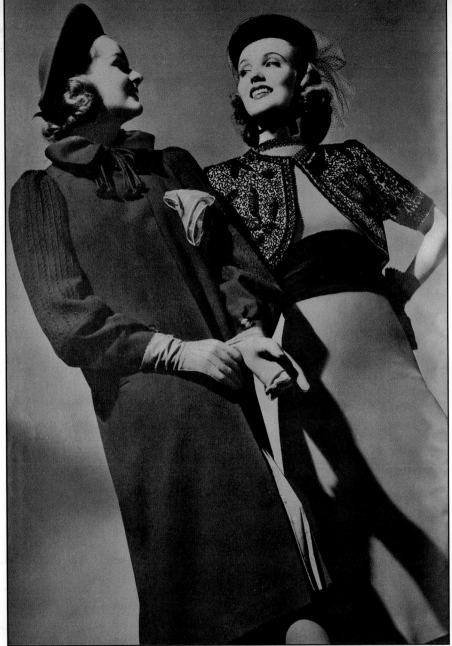

This boxy swagger is without a doubt the smartest coat of the season in Botany All Wool Worsted with full novelty tucked sleeves, folded flower-petal collar with smart ties, and lined with finer quality weighted Silk Crepe. Bolero dress is the number one new fashion of the season with narrow Soutache braid in all-over design, braid outlines the soft, high neckline of the dress, a wide draped cummerbund girdle accents the midriff, and has zip closing from neck to waist at back and side placket.
Spring/Summer 1938

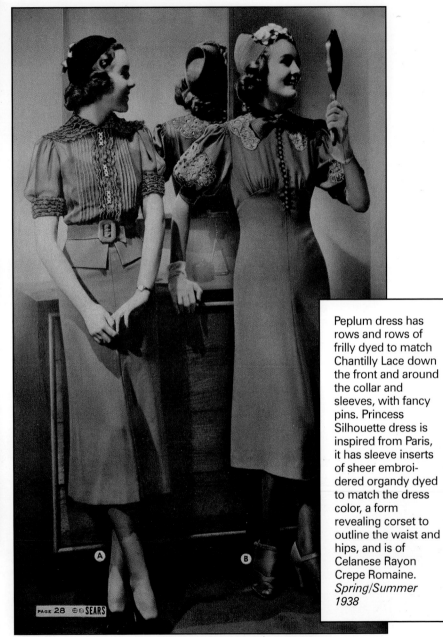

Peplum dress has rows and rows of frilly dyed to match Chantilly Lace down the front and around the collar and sleeves, with fancy pins. Princess Silhouette dress is inspired from Paris, it has sleeve inserts of sheer embroidered organdy dyed to match the dress color, a form revealing corset to outline the waist and hips, and is of Celanese Rayon Crepe Romaine.
Spring/Summer 1938

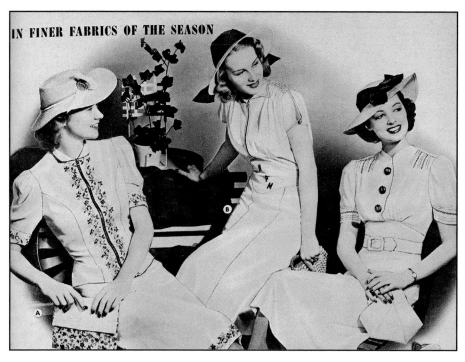

IN FINER FABRICS OF THE SEASON

Petit Point Embroidery dress is of the very new fashion with embroidery running around the hem of the skirt, up the front of the blouse and around the sleeve bottoms. Very chic. Initial dress has three initials on the wide shaped corselet belt, in Celanese Rayon Pebble Crepe. Sharkella dress is of Celanese Rayon, smartly simple, with fagotting and tucks at the shoulders and sleeves. *Spring/Summer 1938*

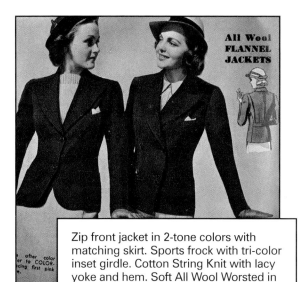

Zip front jacket in 2-tone colors with matching skirt. Sports frock with tri-color inset girdle. Cotton String Knit with lacy yoke and hem. Soft All Wool Worsted in the classic 2-piece style. *Spring/ Summer 1938*

Stunning frock with exquisite hand drawn work on the sleeves, has a roll collar that gives a slenderizing effect, in smooth Celanese Rayon Crepe Romaine. Redingote suit with coat and bright print dress in a smart style. *Spring/Summer 1938*

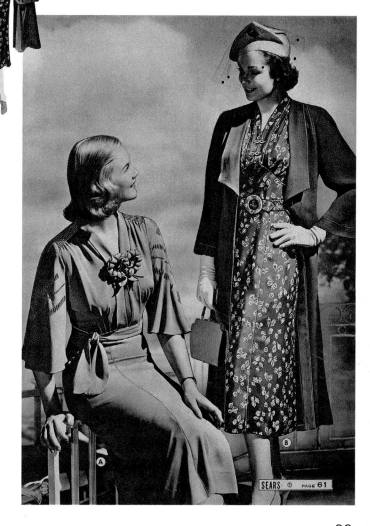

33

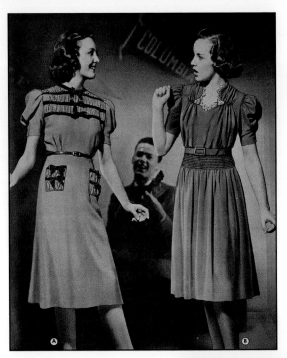

Going Places dresses for juniors in styles that feature bows, sweetheart neck-lines, and pleats. *Fall/Winter 1938/1939*

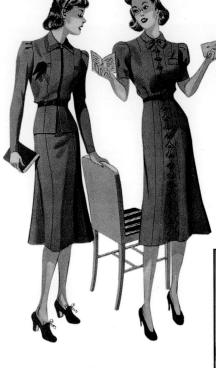

2-piece dress of Spun Rayon Flannel in short or long sleeves, crown zip front closing, with a bright hankie included. Tailored Spun Rayon and Wool "Hopsacking" dress with scallops and contrasting buttons and belt. A "Campus Classic" jumper dress in all wool flannel has detachable suspenders. "Scene-Shifter" dress for mixing and matching has fan pleated skirt and tweed jacket. *Fall/Winter 1938/1939*

"Birthday Girl" dress fastens with birthstone studs, peter pan collar, and pleated fluting. "Dual Personality" is a one-piece dress that can be worn with or without the embroidered jacket. Frock has Celanese Rayon Taffeta on puff sleeves and bias cut skirt, with sparkling metal buttons from the peter pan collar to the V of the fitted bodice. *Fall/Winter 1938/1939*

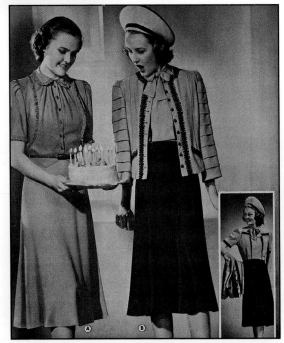

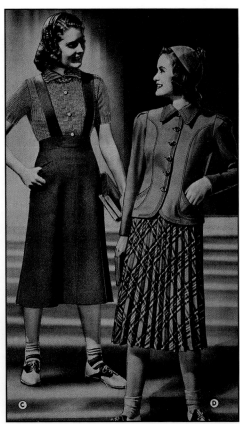

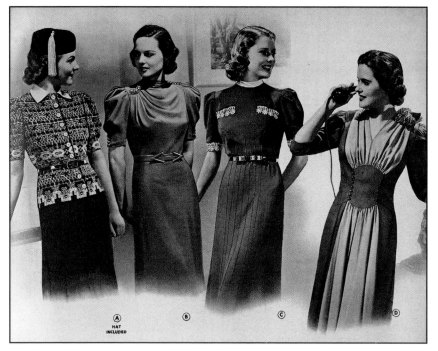

(A) (B) (C) (D)
HAT INCLUDED

2-piece effect dress is made of Celanese Rayon Pebble Crepe, has all-over embroidery, and comes with a "Bell-Hop" hat with tassels to match the embroidery. Flattering dress in Satin-Back Celanese Rayon Crepe Amigo has a draped neckline that closes on the shoulder with buttons and loops. Lovely Celanese Rayon Satin Black Crepe Amigo with white lace medallion edging on pockets and cuffs. Inspired by Alix, famous French designer, this gorgeous dress is of Celanese Rayon Pebble Crepe and has shirred top and apron-front panels. *Fall/Winter 1938/1939*

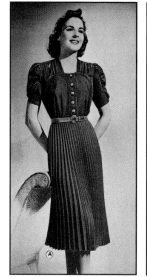
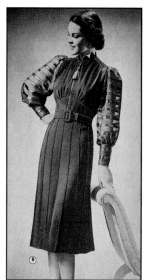

(A) (B)

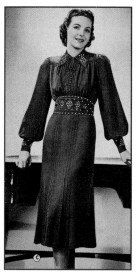
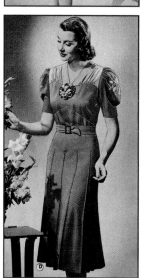

(C) (D)

New fall dresses in Celanese Rayon Pebble Crepe fabric with "Rain-Away" to resist water spots. *Fall/Winter 1938/1939*

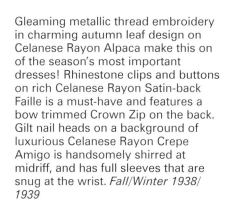

Gleaming metallic thread embroidery in charming autumn leaf design on Celanese Rayon Alpaca make this on of the season's most important dresses! Rhinestone clips and buttons on rich Celanese Rayon Satin-back Faille is a must-have and features a bow trimmed Crown Zip on the back. Gilt nail heads on a background of luxurious Celanese Rayon Crepe Amigo is handsomely shirred at midriff, and has full sleeves that are snug at the wrist. *Fall/Winter 1938/1939*

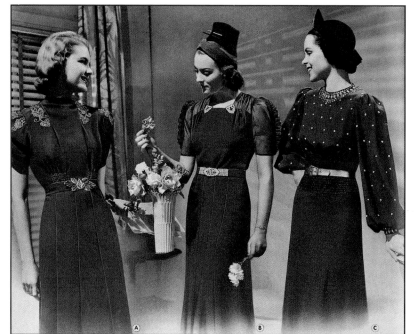

(A) (B) (C)

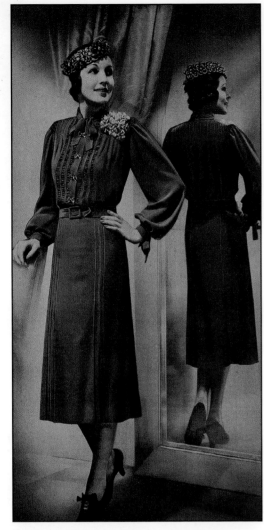

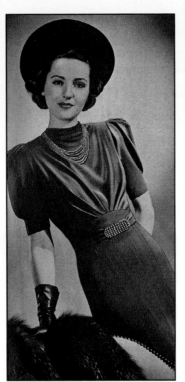

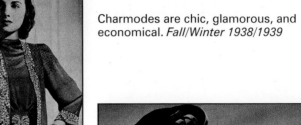

Charmodes are chic, glamorous, and economical. *Fall/Winter 1938/1939*

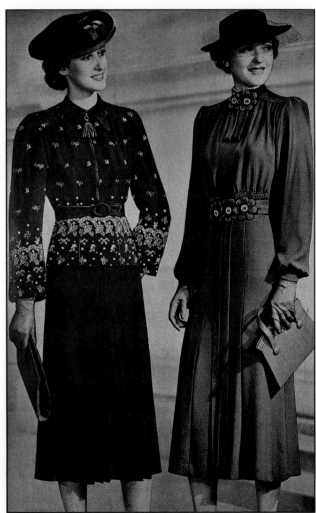

The Anne Williams dress for Fall 1938. Fashion Crepe, a superior-quality Celanese Rayon Crepe has a richly pebbled surface and a gleaming Satin-back. Daintily shirred, with glass buttons, this dress looks so smart. *Fall/Winter 1938/1939*

Colorful Charmodes have Persian-styled embroidery on sleeves and bottom of over blouse, and Soutache braid medallions with novelty centers. Both made of Satin Back Crepe Amigo of Celanese Rayon. *Fall/Winter 1938/1939*

Frock with smocked bodice, V-neck line studded with a pin, and self belt with bow. Lacy, frost-white lingerie, twelve neat buttons, two pert little pockets and kerchief give this frock a lot of young dash. Occasion Dress has dyed-to-match lace on collar, shoulders, and arms. *Fall/Winter 1938/1939*

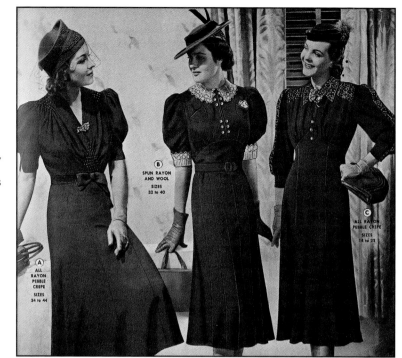

Satin Back Celanese rayon Faille dress has smart scroll trimming from neck to hem, sleeves that tie, and novelty pin and bow. *Fall/Winter 1938/1939*

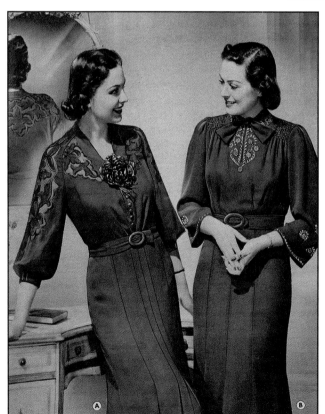

Smart, youthful dresses of All Rayon Pebble Crepe and Spun Rayon challis fabrics. *Fall/Winter 1938/1939*

Latest version of the "Appliqué Dress" made of Rayon Crepe, silk chiffon appliqué on yoke that extends to the bracelet sleeves. Beauvais embroidery and nail heads adorn this dress with new loose bracelet sleeves, high-tie collar, and flared skirt. *Fall/Winter 1938/1939*

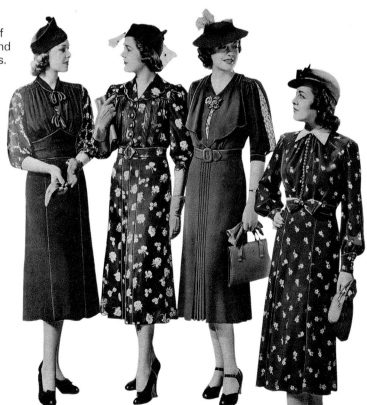

37

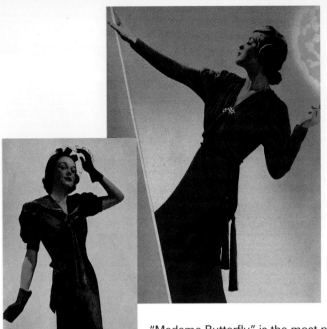

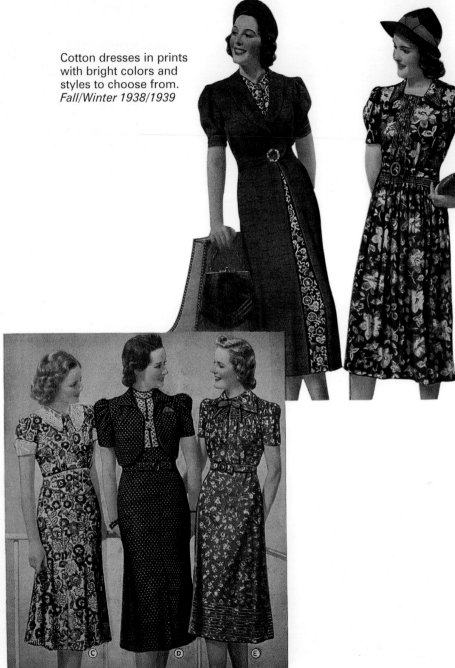

Cotton dresses in prints with bright colors and styles to choose from. *Fall/Winter 1938/1939*

"Madame Butterfly" is the most popular date-and dance frock in crisp, rustling Taffeta and appliquéd all over with brilliant "petit point" butterflies! "Glamour Girl" is designed by America's leading designer, Elinor Weems, is sleek and slim with shirred bosom and swirling skirt. A new silhouette has the feminine grace that men adore with a slender waistline, and bright embroidery. Gold gilt nail heads adorn this glittering bodice and is made of Pebble Crepe of Celanese. *Fall/Winter 1937-1938*

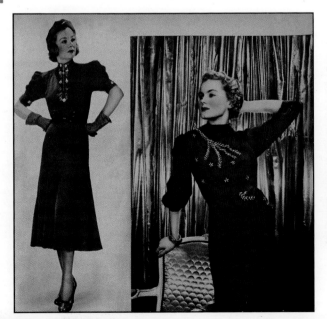

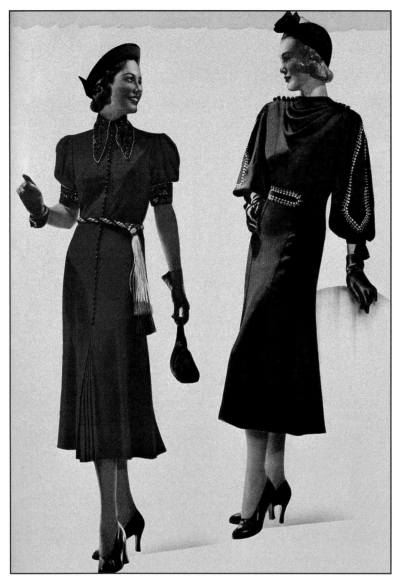

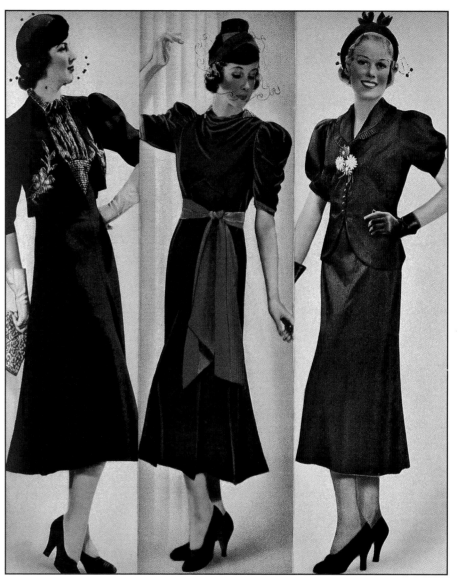

Marietta Crepe of Celanese two-piece dress with saddle stitching is beautifully hand-worked in rich rayon floss to match ascot scarf. Pebble Crepe of Celanese Princess lined flared skirt with brilliant peasant bandings. Persian-type embroidery on Satin-back Crepe Amigo of Celanese, and peplum is embroidered all around. Marietta Crepe of Celanese dress has richly embroidered collar, Tyrolean cord girdle and tassel. Pebble Crepe of Celanese dress with flattering cowl neckline, big sleeves, and gilded nail head studding. *Fall/Winter 1937-1938*

Bolero effect dress with glittering metal Lame on Satin-back Crepe Amigo of Celanese. Dress of Transparent Velvet is silk-backed with rayon pile, has 2-tone girdle, and lovely sleeve bandings of sheer Chiffon. Celanese Taffeta 2-piece style dress has knife pleating on collar, and nosegay of field flowers for color accent. *Fall/Winter 1937-1938*

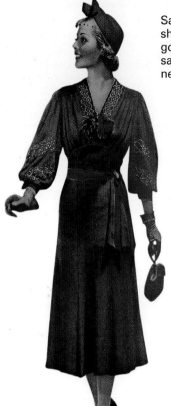

Satin Back Faille dress has fine shirring at the shoulders, skirt is gored for a light swing, 2-tone sash, and big flowers at the neckline. *Fall/Winter 1937-1938*

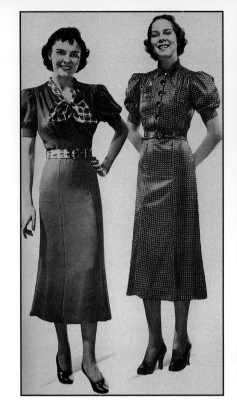

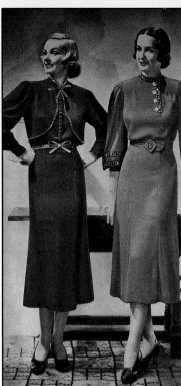

Dresses of Pebble Crepe Taffeta trim, polka dot rayon taffeta, gay young bolero style, and embroidered trim are all flattering and priced low! *Fall/Winter 1937-1938*

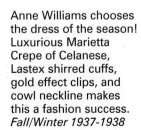

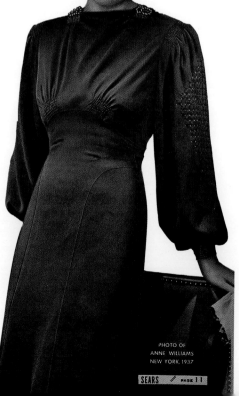

Anne Williams chooses the dress of the season! Luxurious Marietta Crepe of Celanese, Lastex shirred cuffs, gold effect clips, and cowl neckline makes this a fashion success. *Fall/Winter 1937-1938*

PHOTO OF
ANNE WILLIAMS
NEW YORK, 1937

SEARS / PAGE 11

Trimline fashion dresses in transparent velvet and embroidered Pebble Crepe of Celanese makes larger women look their loveliest. *Fall/Winter 1937-1938*

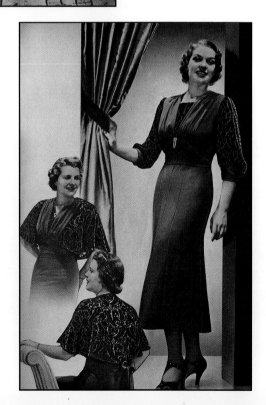

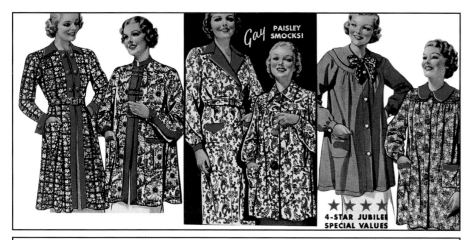

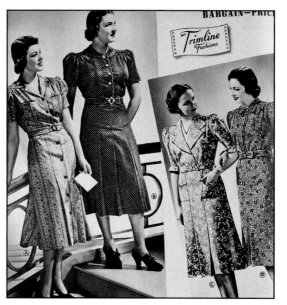

Shirtwaist dress has button-down front, shirred shoulders, and high pockets. Dress made of Percale has white polka dots, scalloped collar, and down bodice front. Monotone Print dress lingerie trim on pockets and sleeves, and a white vestee. Long sleeved Flannelette is one-piece, Crown zip front, and a 2" hem. *Fall/Winter 1939-1940*

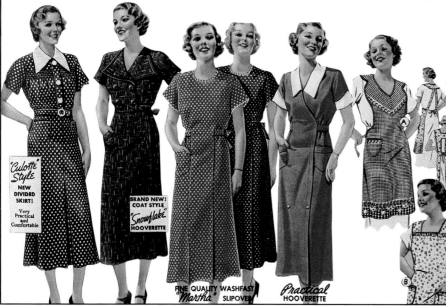

A variety of smocks, slipovers, and aprons. *Fall/Winter 1936-1937*

Windbreaker style blouse has collarless neckline and wide snug waist. plaid skirt has all around pleating and two-button waist closing, All Wool Tweed jacket with handsome wide stripes with bright contrasting nubs, and 4-gore flare skirt is All Wool Flannel. *Fall/Winter 1939-1940*

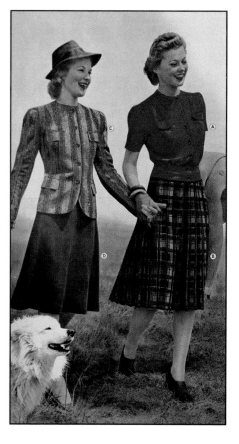

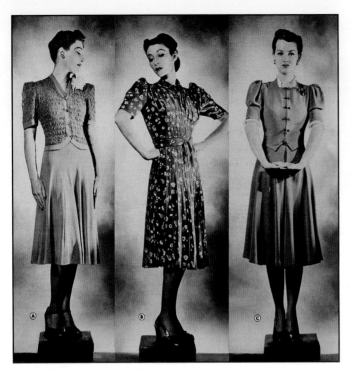

Sail Along print dresses in vibrant, new, Luxable colors are made of Spun Rayon, and Spun Rayon with Silk Noil. *Spring/Summer 1939*

Waffle shirred Jacket Dress, blouse of silk chiffon with rayon taffeta bodice, skirt made of Celanese Rayon Crepe Romaine. Prints and pleats dress is made of Celanese Rayon Crepe Romaine, in gorgeous colors destined to make you look pretty as a picture. 2-piece dress of Celanese Rayon Crepe Romaine or Celanese Rayon Taffeta for a quaint and fashionable new look. *Spring/Summer 1939*

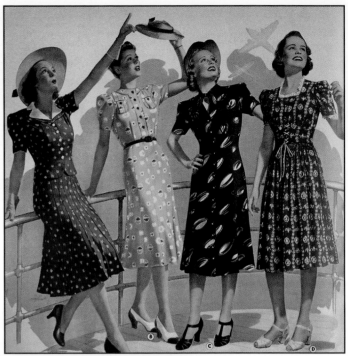

New print dresses, worn with flowers, are a perfect choice when you want to be "dressed" but not "dinner dressed". In a variety of colors and styles, these dresses are a truly smart solution for the modern woman. *Spring/Summer 1939*

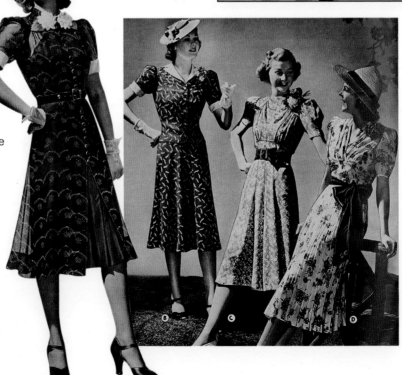

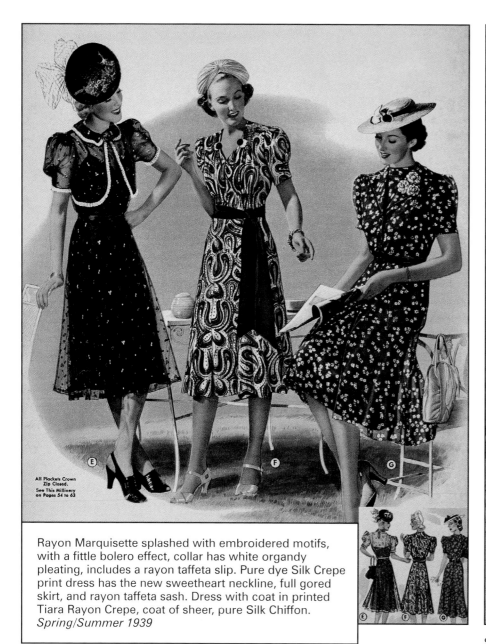

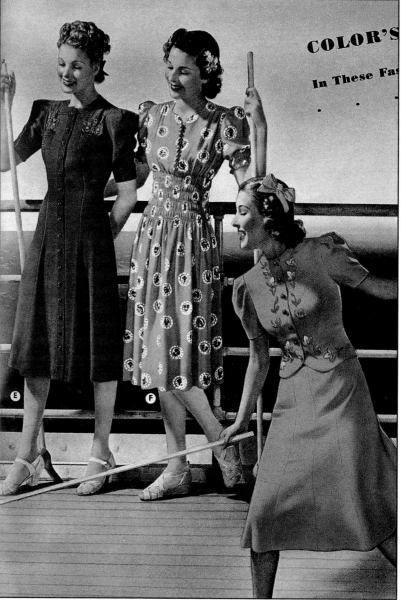

Rayon Marquisette splashed with embroidered motifs, with a fittle bolero effect, collar has white organdy pleating, includes a rayon taffeta slip. Pure dye Silk Crepe print dress has the new sweetheart neckline, full gored skirt, and rayon taffeta sash. Dress with coat in printed Tiara Rayon Crepe, coat of sheer, pure Silk Chiffon. *Spring/Summer 1939*

Schiaparelli's high flowerpot pockets in gay embroidery, buttons from neck to hem, and rows of stitching down the front. Dirndl dress has shirred midriff with Latex thread, new sweetheart neckline, and shrug shoulders. Two-piece dress is broad shouldered, has basque-waisted jacket embroidered in bright wools and fastened with gay buttons, cardigan neckline, and gored to flare gently. All dresses are of good quality Spun Rayon *Sail Along* Luxable colors. *Spring/Summer 1939*

43

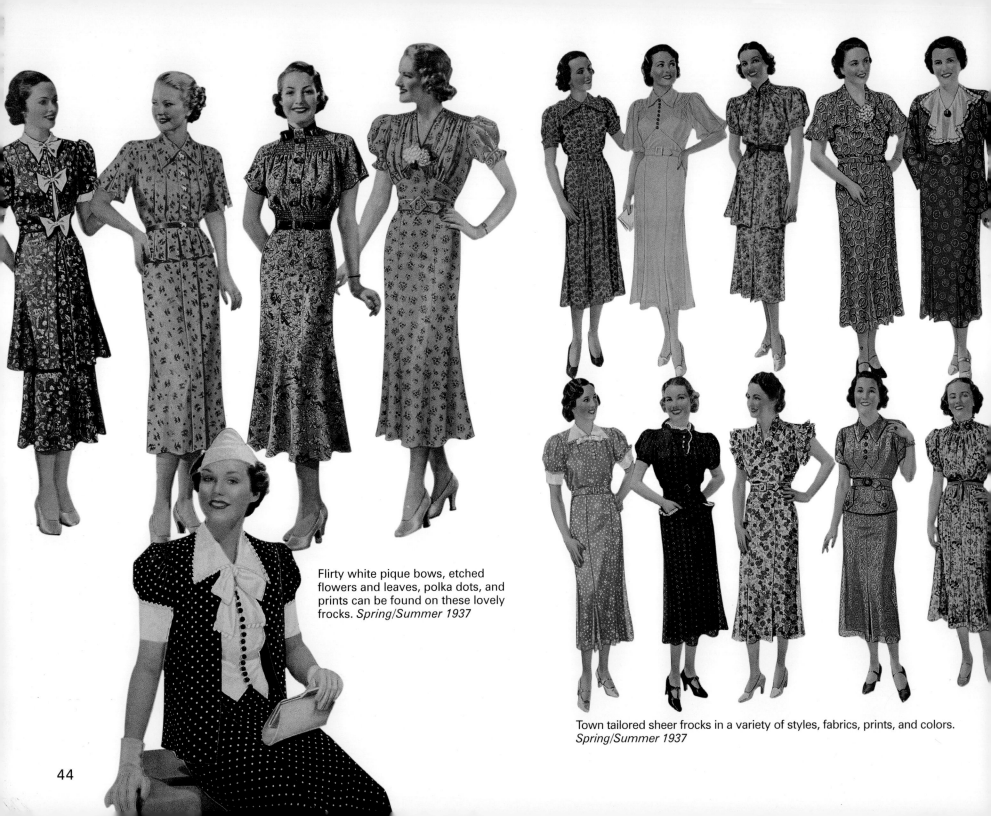

Flirty white pique bows, etched flowers and leaves, polka dots, and prints can be found on these lovely frocks. *Spring/Summer 1937*

Town tailored sheer frocks in a variety of styles, fabrics, prints, and colors. *Spring/Summer 1937*

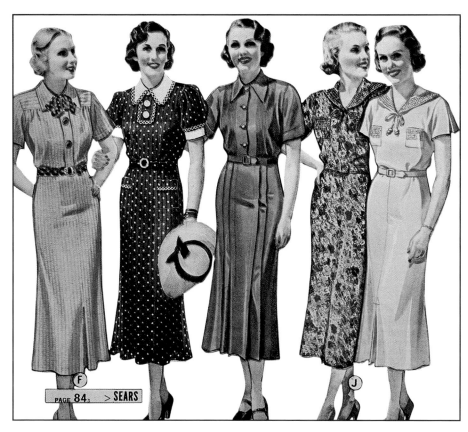

Dresses that give your figure a slenderizing effect for the modern woman.
Spring/Summer 1937

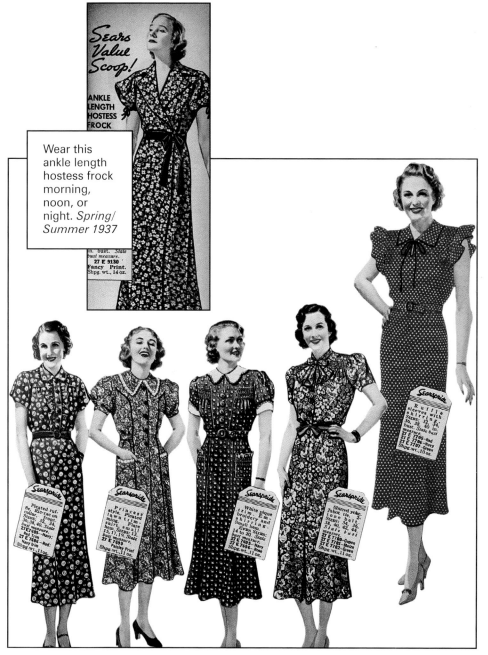

Sears
Value
Scoop!

ANKLE
LENGTH
HOSTESS
FROCK

Wear this
ankle length
hostess frock
morning,
noon, or
night. *Spring/
Summer 1937*

Percale dresses in the latest styles and newest prints. Full cut, 2" hems.
Spring/Summer 1937

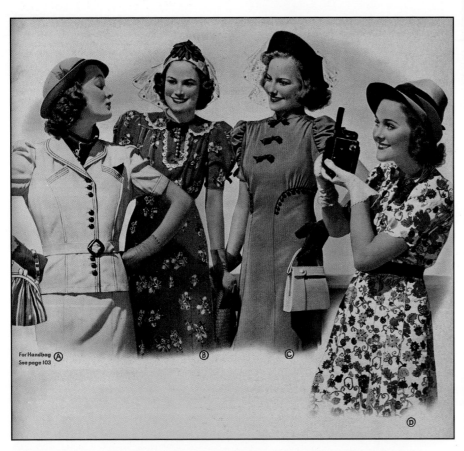

2-piece dress in soft colors on Bengaline Cotton. Flower Basket Print dress in Crown Tested Tiara French-type Rayon Crepe. Corselet dress in glorious colors on Celanese Rayon Pebble Crepe. Sun-Shan print on Crown Tested Spun Rayon. *Spring/Summer 1938*

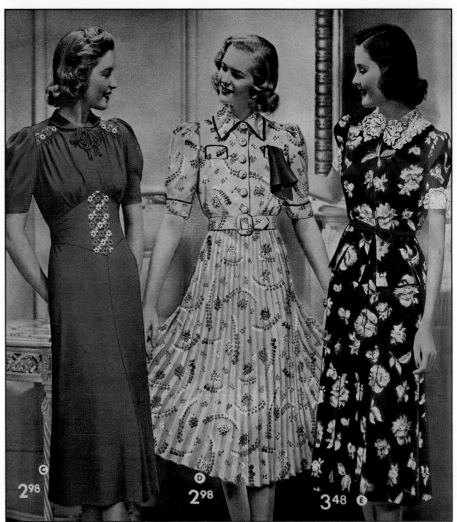

Dresses with high necklines, slim fitting waistlines, colorful accents, pleated skirts, and new prints. Lovely. *Spring/Summer 1938*

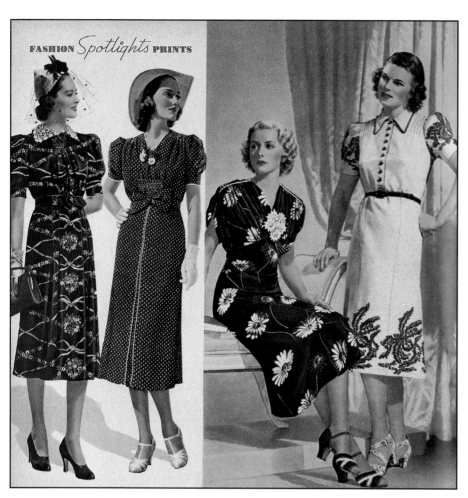

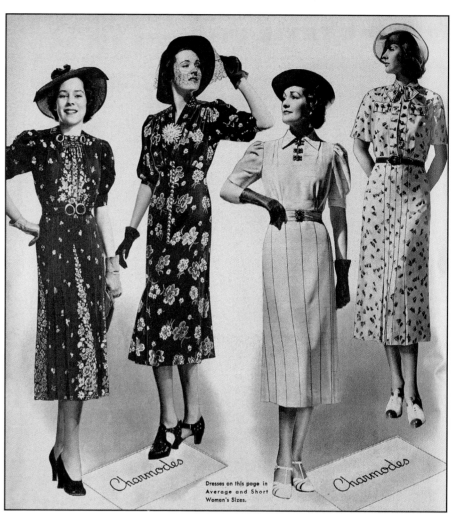

Bow Knot Panel Print dress with detachable lace collar. Crown Tested Rayon French Type Crepe dress with pin dot pattern. Zip dress has zips at the shoulders and another closes the placket, new corselet waist, and a corsage of daisies. Dress with intricate design embroidery, definitely 1938 styling. *Spring/Summer 1938*

Charmodes in gorgeous prints and shantung styles. *Spring/Summer 1938*

All Wool skirt with umbrella tucks all around. Skirt with cluster pleats at front, kick-pleat in back. Sharkskin skirt has two double kick-pleats at front, single pleat in back. Cotton Twill skirt has long zip fasteners. Plaid or plain skirt with slits on each side. Flannel skirt is well tailored with three pleats in front with a panel back. *Spring/Summer 1938*

Phillis frocks are of finest quality percale, Sanforized-shrunk, with gay sparkling prints in all the latest fashions. *Spring/Summer 1938*

Good News are for women who wear a larger size who want a slenderizing effect. These dresses are flattering and smart. *Fall/Winter 1938/1939*

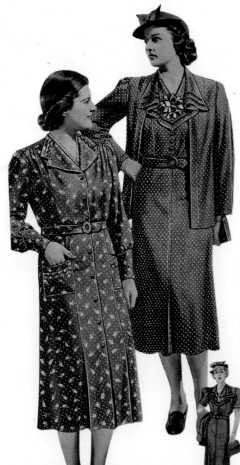

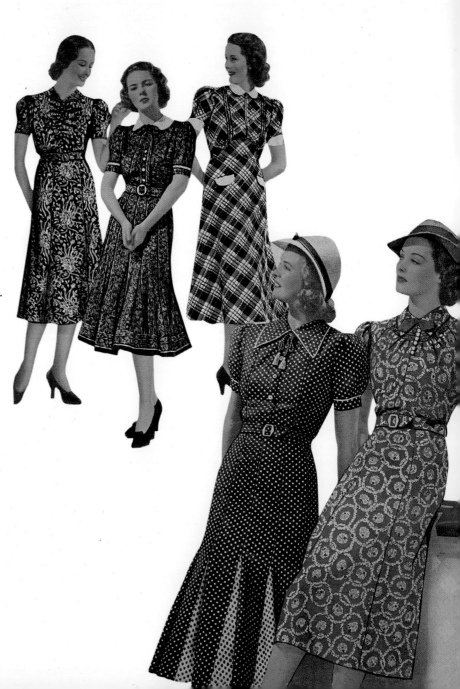

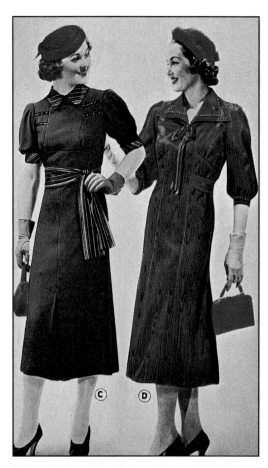

"French Room" frocks in styles and fabrics that are so smart and new, you will want two! *Fall/Winter 1937-1938*

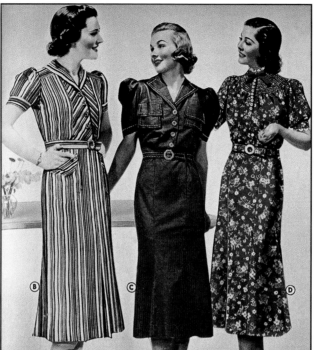

Daytime frocks are a four star feature in floral prints, stripes, solids with contrasting saddle-stitching, and paisley patterns. *Fall/Winter 1937-1938*

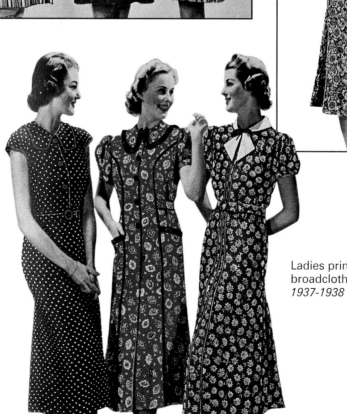

Ladies print frocks on percales and broadcloths in many styles. *Fall/Winter 1937-1938*

Maternity Dresses

Aprons

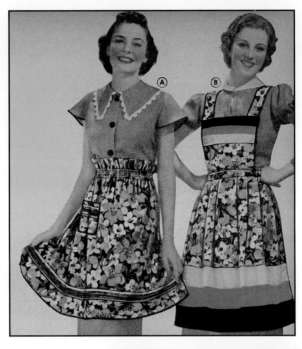

Tyrolean aprons in quaint styles that will brighten your day at home. *Fall/Winter 1937-1938*

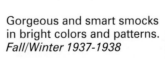

Maternity dresses are adjustable to every figure change, come in small pretty prints, and are designed for comfort. *Spring/Summer 1938*

Gorgeous and smart smocks in bright colors and patterns. *Fall/Winter 1937-1938*

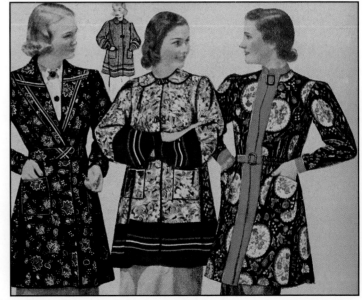

Sweaters/Blouses

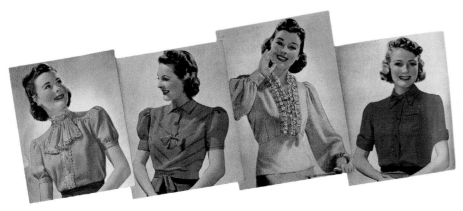

Blouses that come in paisley prints, with jabots, harmonized stitching, bishop sleeves, All Silk Crepe, Rayon Satin or Sheer, feminine frills, Rayon Satin stripes, or buttons galore. *Fall/Winter 1939-1940*

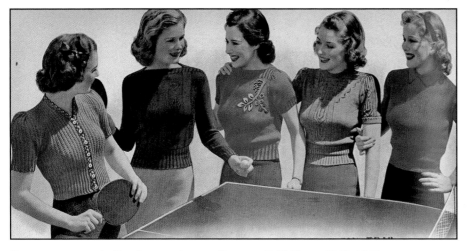

Sporty sweaters in Cardigan styles or slip-ons. *Fall/Winter 1939-1940*

All wool worsted "Twins" sweaters in rust, royal blue, and bright red colors. *Fall/Winter 1937-1938*

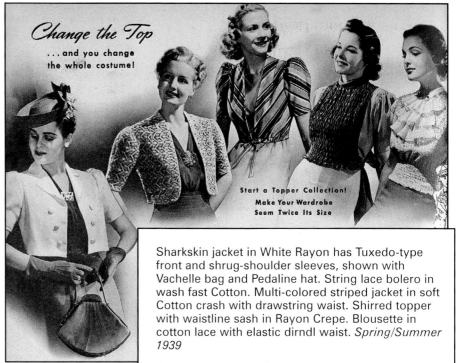

Change the Top
...and you change the whole costume!

Start a Topper Collection! Make Your Wardrobe Seem Twice Its Size

Sharkskin jacket in White Rayon has Tuxedo-type front and shrug-shoulder sleeves, shown with Vachelle bag and Pedaline hat. String lace bolero in wash fast Cotton. Multi-colored striped jacket in soft Cotton crash with drawstring waist. Shirred topper with waistline sash in Rayon Crepe. Blousette in cotton lace with elastic dirndl waist. *Spring/Summer 1939*

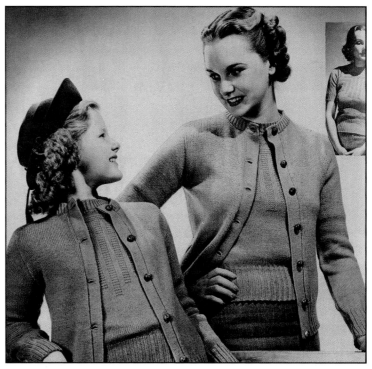

Sportswear

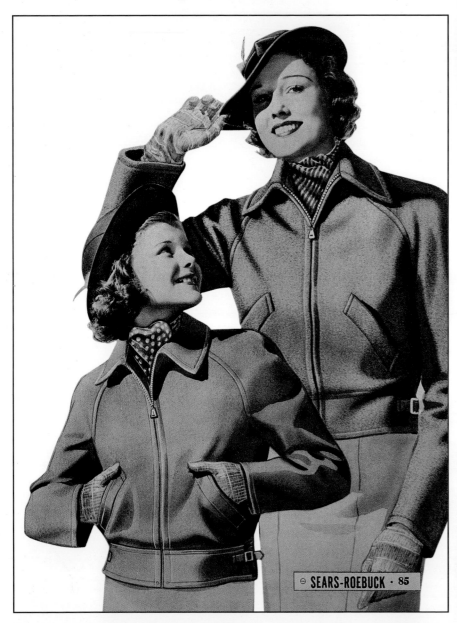

Cossack style jackets in Cotton Suede Cloth, Genuine Suede-Tex, or All Wool have adjustable buckles for a snug fit, and zipper closing. *Fall/Winter 1936-1937*

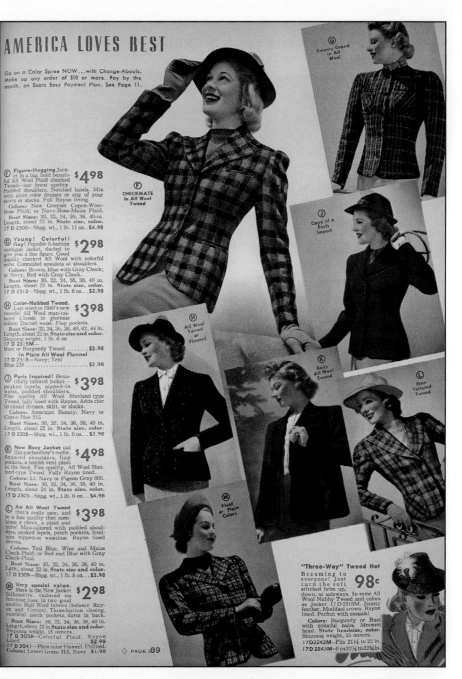

Change-about jackets in a wide assortment of colors and styles. *Fall/Winter 1939-1940*

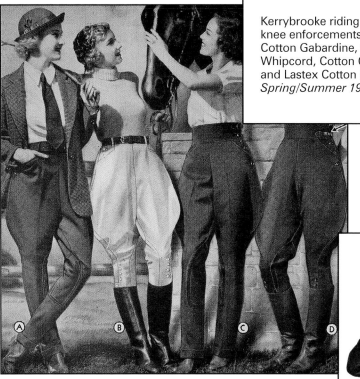

Kerrybrooke riding togs with knee enforcements come in Cotton Gabardine, Cotton Whipcord, Cotton Cavalry Twill, and Lastex Cotton Cavalry Twill. *Spring/Summer 1937*

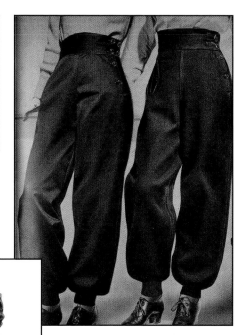

Ski pants with new built-up waist bands in cotton gabardine, wool, and heavy Melton fabrics. *Fall/Winter 1937-1938*

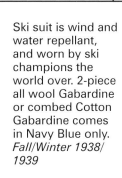

Ski suit is wind and water repellant, and worn by ski champions the world over. 2-piece all wool Gabardine or combed Cotton Gabardine comes in Navy Blue only. *Fall/Winter 1938/1939*

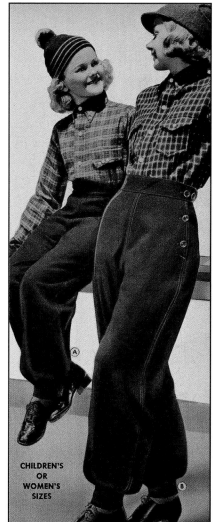

CHILDREN'S OR WOMEN'S SIZES

Ski pants are water repellent wool, full-cut, double stitched, with adjustable Ski-Slide fasteners. *Fall/Winter 1937-1938*

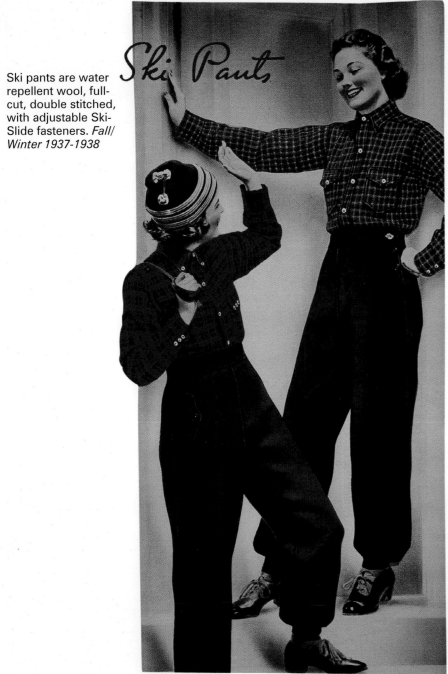

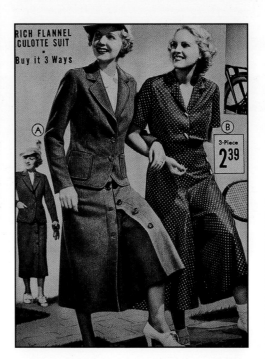

"Two-Timer" flannel Culotte suit for street or play, when button looks like a tailored skirt, unbuttoned gives the freedom of trousers. Polka Dot Cotton Pongette, with shorts and blouse. *Spring/Summer 1937*

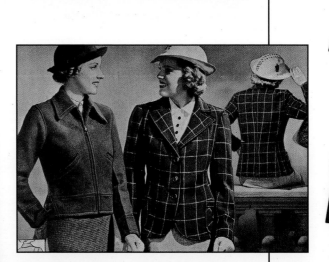

Give your wardrobe a sporty look with a fine wool Cossack, plaid jacket, Gabardine sport suit, All Wool Jersey, or Checked coat with All Wool flannel skirt. *Spring/Summer 1937*

PJs, Robes and Loungewear

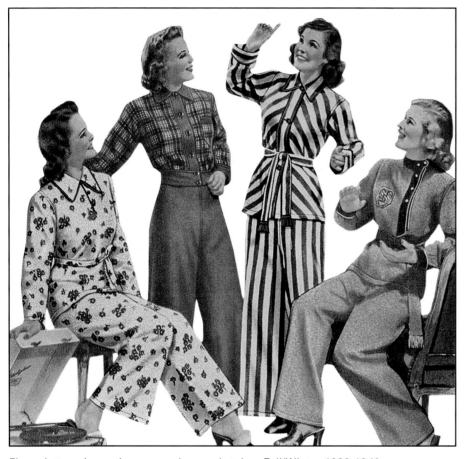

Flannelette pajamas in many colors and styles. *Fall/Winter 1939-1940*

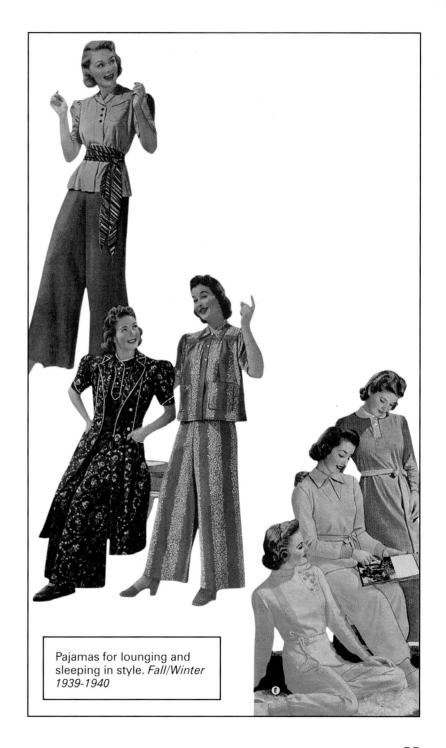

Pajamas for lounging and sleeping in style. *Fall/Winter 1939-1940*

Tailored 2-piece pajama sets in Peasant Cotton Print, Broad-cloth, Checked Cotton Print, and sheer Floral Batiste. *Spring/Summer 1939*

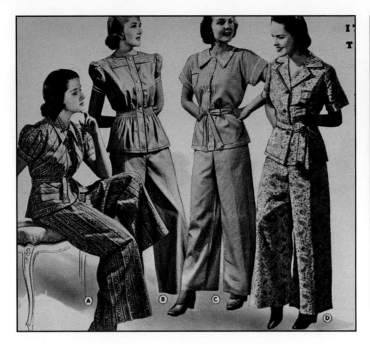

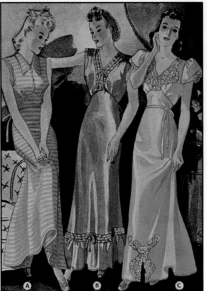

Sleepwear in shimmering striped rayon gowns, print pajamas with matching quilted jacket, spun rayon and cotton gown, and man tailored styles. *Fall/Winter 1939-1940*

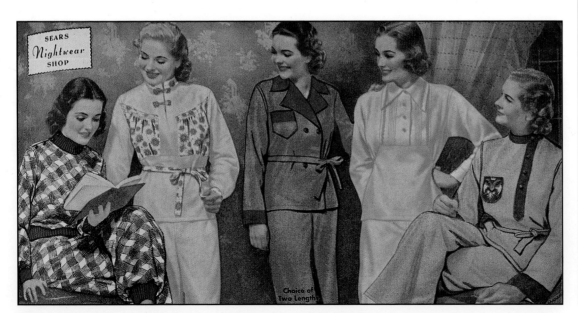

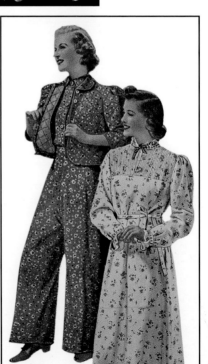

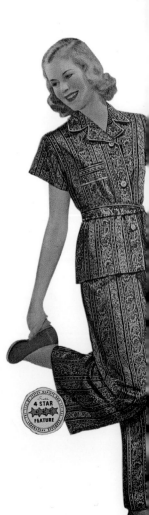

Flannelette pajamas and gowns give chill-defying comfort in solids and prints. *Fall/Winter 1938/1939*

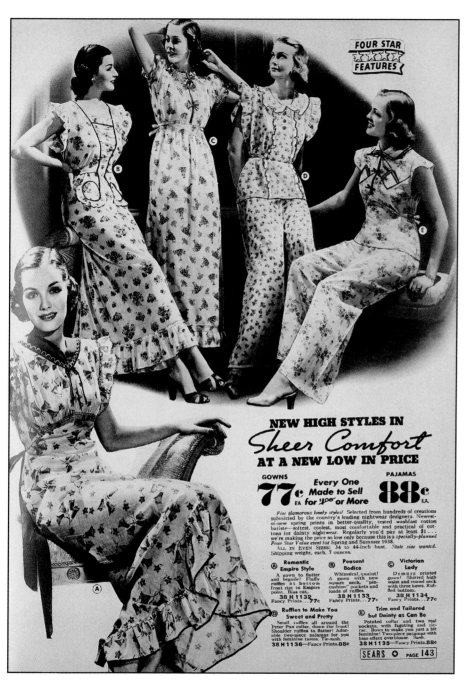

Sheer Comfort nightgowns and pajamas in five glamorous styles and prints. *Spring/Summer 1938*

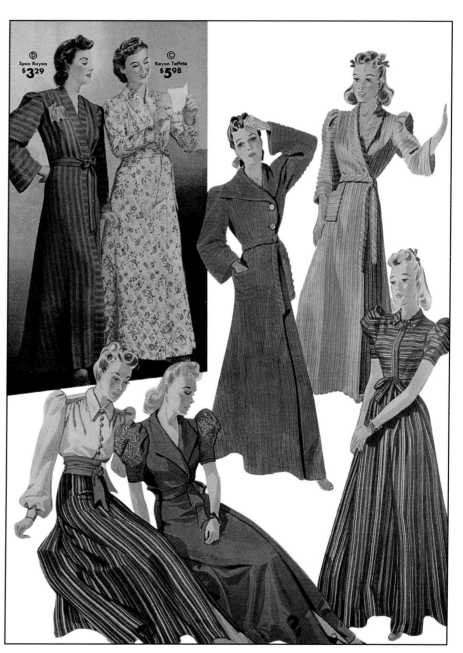

Oh so warm housecoats come in rayon taffeta, spun rayon, cotton chenille, slub cotton, and Rayon French-type Crepe fabrics. *Fall/Winter 1939-1940*

Loungewear and robes in rich warm corduroy, fluffy soft rayon fleece, all wool flannel, and rayon satin. *Fall/Winter 1938/1939*

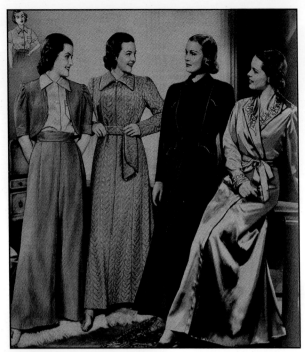

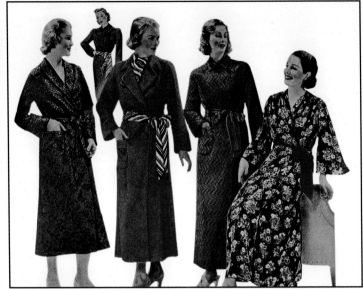

Balbriggans give soft and cozy comfort in styles such as shirt-style gowns, striped top with plain trousers, two-piece pajamas with crew neck, and Russian-style blouse. *Fall/Winter 1937-1938*

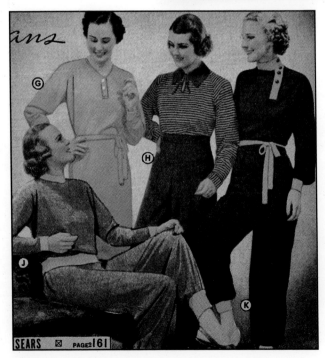

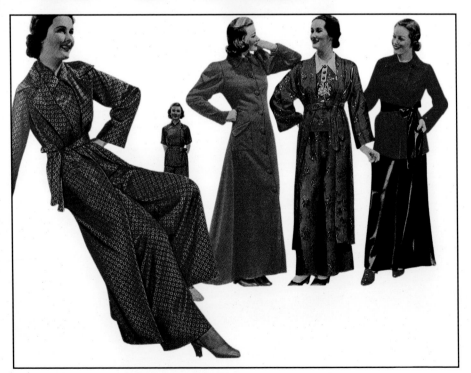

Lovely robes, 2-piece lounge suits, and 3-piece pajama ensemble offer every woman a variety of styles and colors. *Fall/Winter 1937-1938*

Lingerie

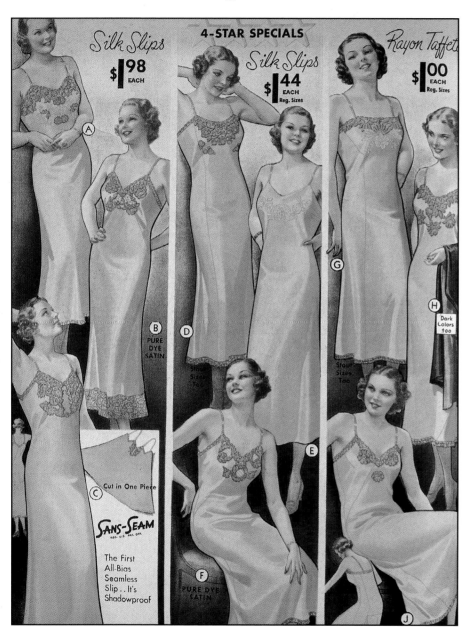

Luxurious silk or rayon bias cut slips. *Fall/Winter 1936-1937*

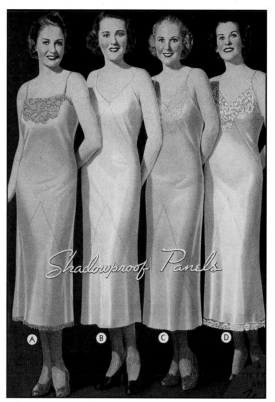

Silk slips with bodice top in lace trim, tailored style double front, tailored and embroidered, and California lace trimmed top. *Spring/Summer 1937*

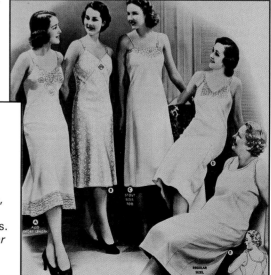

Rayon Taffeta slips with wide lace bottoms, shadow prints, bodice top/shadow panels, and straight front/bias backs. *Spring/Summer 1938*

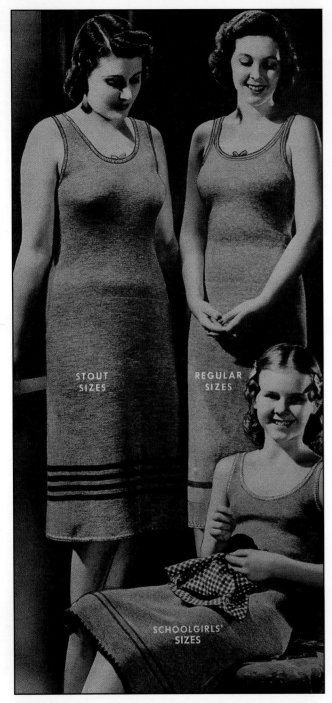

STOUT SIZES

REGULAR SIZES

SCHOOLGIRLS' SIZES

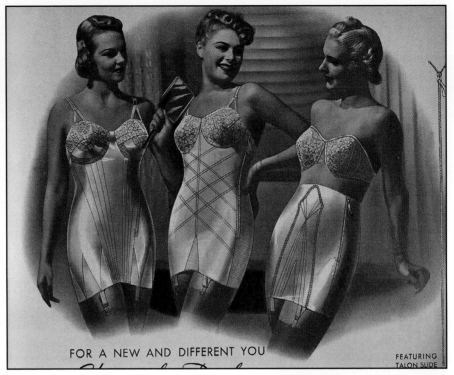

FOR A NEW AND DIFFERENT YOU

FEATURING TALON SLIDE

Charmode Darleen figure controlling girdles features Talon Slide fasteners for faster and smoother closing. Tearose. *Spring/Summer 1939*

The pathway to slenderness starts with a slenderizing girdle. *Spring/Summer 1938*

Knit slips designed to hug your figure snugly for school-girls, and women's regular and stout sizes. *Fall/Winter 1938/1939*

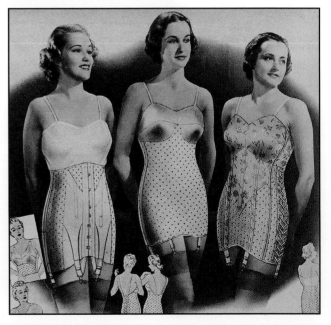

Darleen and Knit Power Net elastic panel girdles for figure control. *Fall/Winter 1938/1939*

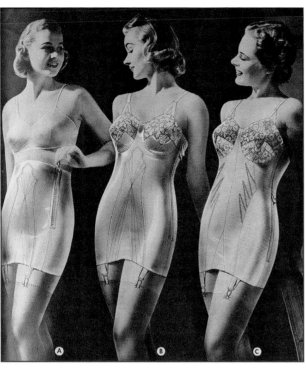

Form fitting support to help your new dresses look their loveliest. *Fall/Winter 1937-1938*

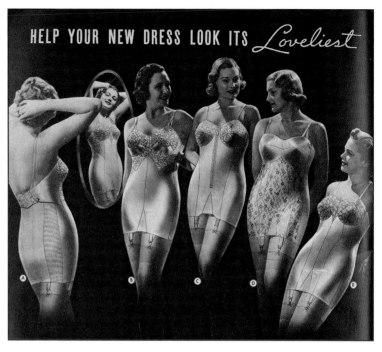

HELP YOUR NEW DRESS LOOK ITS *Loveliest*

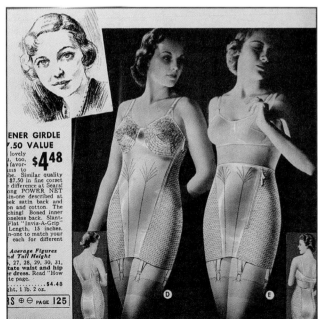

ENER GIRDLE
7.50 VALUE $4.48

lovely
, too,
favor-
ms to
be. Similar quality
$7.50 in fine corset
difference at Sears!
ong POWER NET
in-one described at
eek satin back and
on and cotton. The
ching! Boned inner
oneless back. Slant-
Flat "Inviz-A-Grip"
Length, 15 inches.
n-one to match your
each for different

*Average Figures
nd Tall Height*
, 27, 28, 29, 30, 31,
ate waist and hip
r dress. Read "How
te page.
.........$4.48
ght, 1 lb. 2 oz.

S ⊕ ⊖ PAGE 125

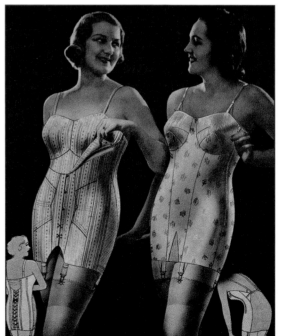

"Bel-Form" girdle has front clasp with side hooking brassiere, and laces at back from waist down. Net-lined rayon jersey has shaped "V" cloth inserts for uplift and elastic back holds down the rear. *Fall/Winter 1937-1938*

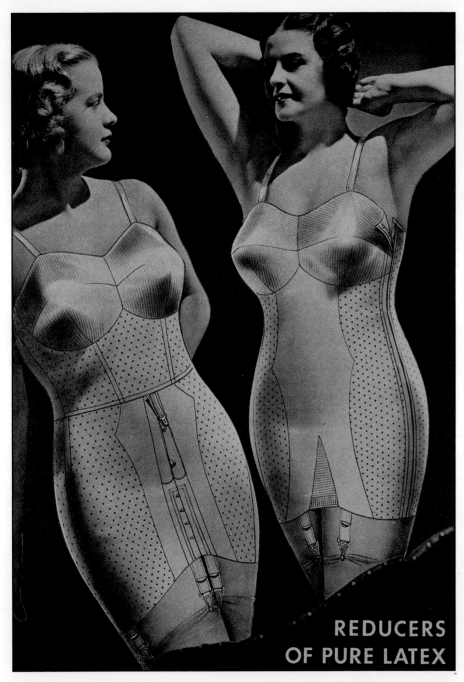

REDUCERS OF PURE LATEX

Pure latex reducing garments slenderize and support your figure. *Fall/Winter 1937-1938*

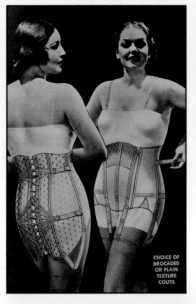

CHOICE OF BROCADED OR PLAIN TEXTURE COUTIL

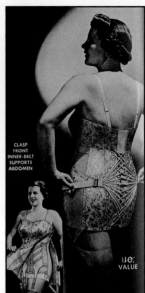

CLASP FRONT INNER-BELT SUPPORTS ABDOMEN

VALUE

Prof-Gale 2-Lace Health belt in your choice of brocaded or plain texture coutil. *Fall/Winter 1937-1938*

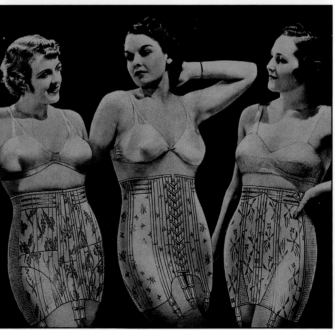

Nu-Back is a four star feature that allows you freedom to stoop, sit, or bend. *Fall/Winter 1937-1938*

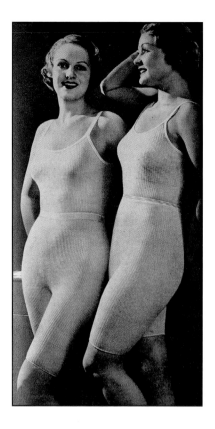 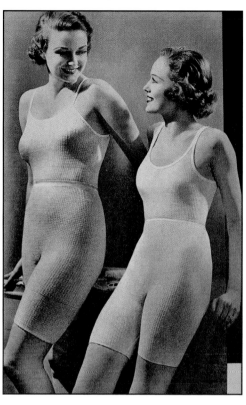

When a gal needs extra warmth she wears "Flatter-ees" vests and panties. *Fall/Winter 1936-1937*

Flatter-ees hide their warmth in beauty. *Fall/Winter 1937-1938*

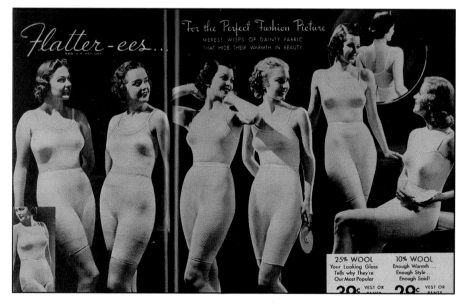

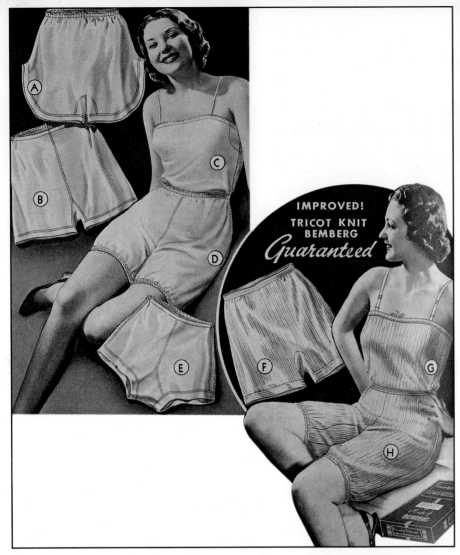

Assorted women's underwear made with quality rayon. *Fall/Winter 1936-1937*

IMPROVED!
TRICOT KNIT
BEMBERG
Guaranteed

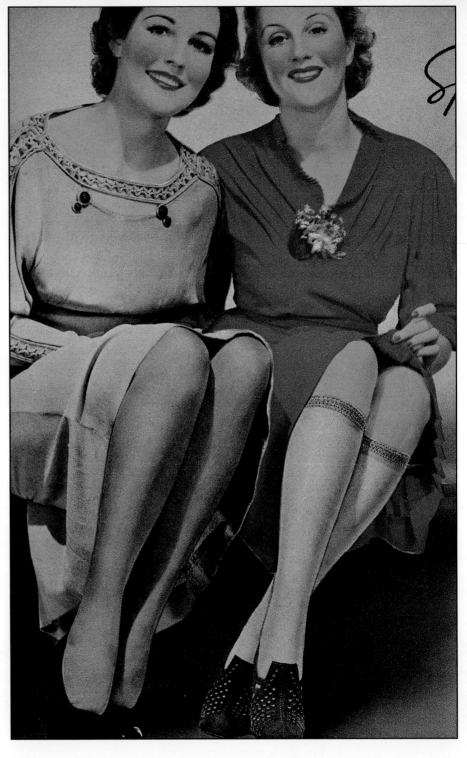

Splash proof silk stockings in knee and regular lengths. *Fall/Winter 1937-1938*

Coats and Suits

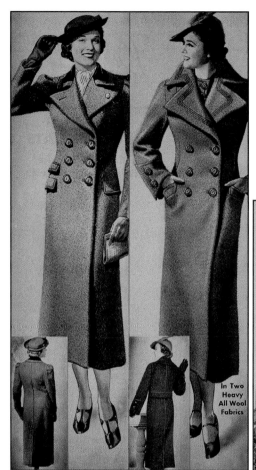

Long wool "Chesterfield", All Wool Melton, All Wool Chinchilla, and 3-piece coat with matching hat and muff with Persian fur fabric. These coats are warm, practical, and stylish. *Fall/Winter 1936-1937*

In Two Heavy All Wool Fabrics

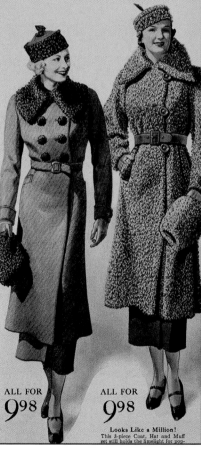

ALL FOR 9⁹⁸   ALL FOR 9⁹⁸

Looks Like a Million!
This 3-piece Coat, Hat and Muff
set still holds the limelight for pop-

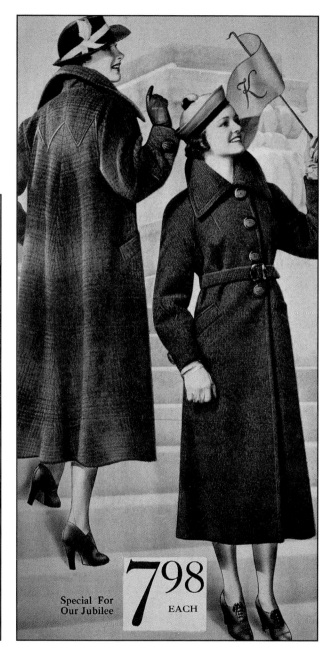

All wool Kerrybrooke sports coats have double-pointed yoke and wide swinging flare, slash pockets, and large buttons. Available in Shadow Plaids or Checked Coating. Length about 47 inches. *Fall/Winter 1936-1937*

Special For Our Jubilee   7⁹⁸ EACH

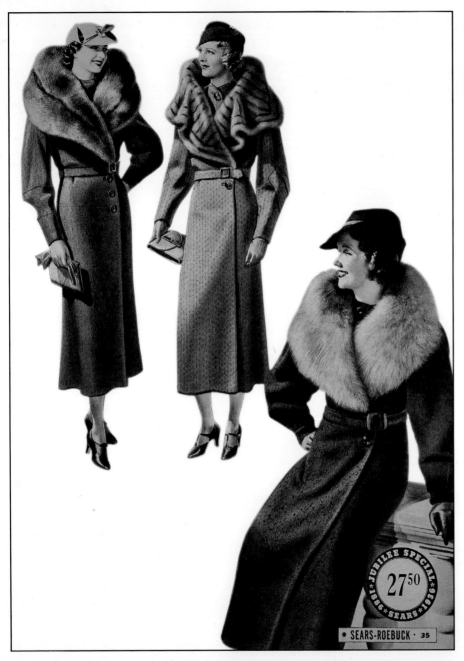

Cortleigh dress coats of all wool genuine Kit Fox, Genuine Mink-Dyed Marmot, and Genuine Marmot have Chamois lining to keep a lady warm. *Fall/Winter 1936-1937*

All coats are genuine Northern buck Coney in your choice of Hudson Seal, Dyed Coney, or Beaver-Dyed Coney. The coat on the left is a Swagger style, on the right is the Semi-Fitted style. *Fall/ Winter*

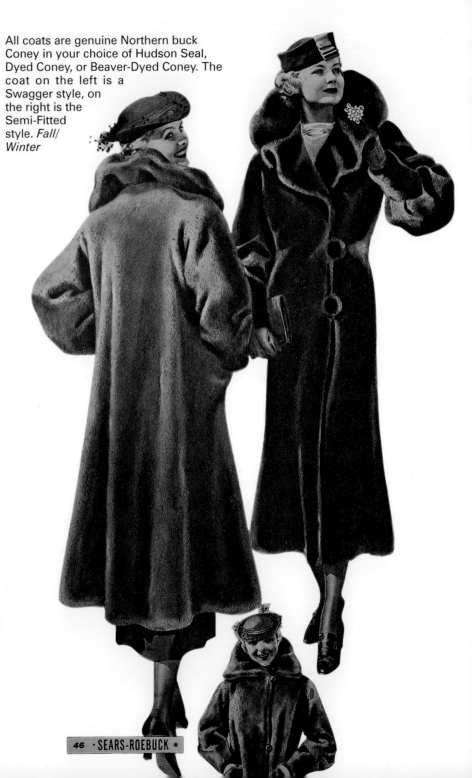

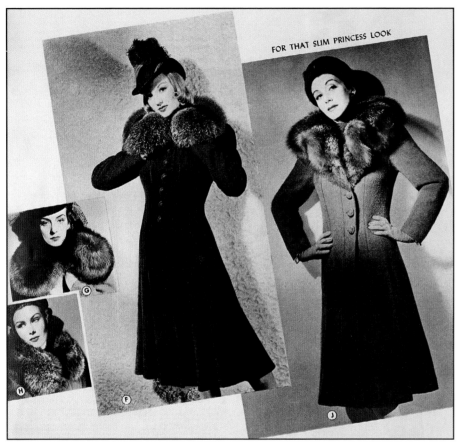

All Wool Boucle tailored in the Princess style with fox fur collars.
Fall/Winter 1939-1940

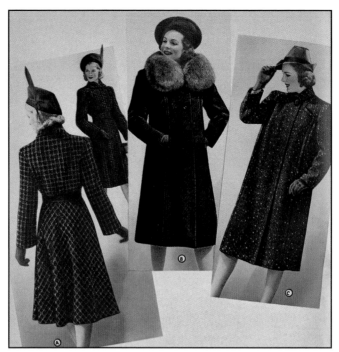

Tweed coats to keep warm come in different styles such as blended plaid that features a "Whirling Dervish" skirt, luxurious raccoon fur collar to flatter your face, and all wool with all new diagonal weave. *Fall/Winter 1939-1940*

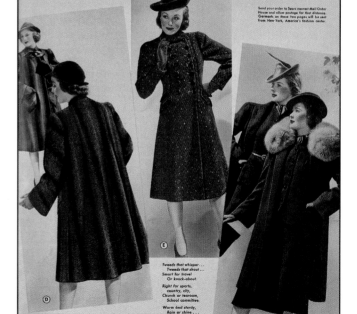

Various Tweed coats in different patterns and styles including a 3-piece wardrobe suit with wolf fur collar. *Fall/Winter 1939-1940*

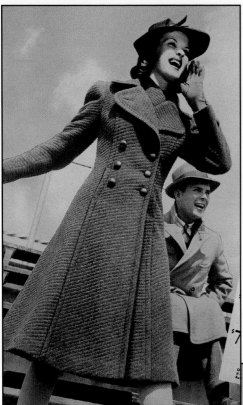

Miss America Polo coat is master tailored with double-breasted reefer lines, molded through the body, flaring at the hem. Square shoulders, dashing wide revers and a stitched slenderizing panel back. *Fall/Winter 1939-1940*

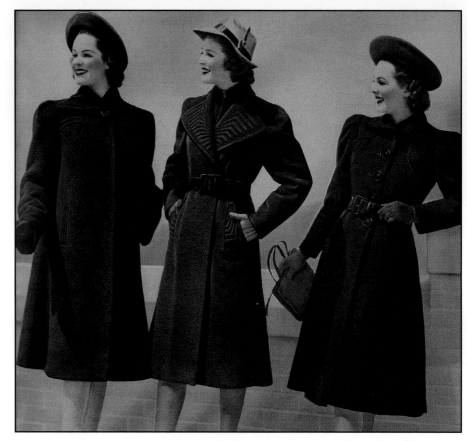

Diagonal weave coat with a square shoulder swagger, new wide revers with trapunto stitching, and a Young Swing silhouette. All wool. *Fall/Winter 1939-1940*

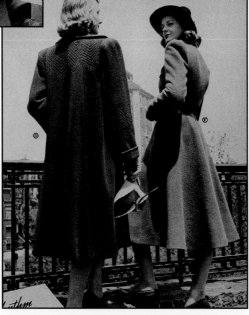

Rippling Rhythm silhouette casual coats in All Wool Fleece. *Fall/ Winter 1939-1940*

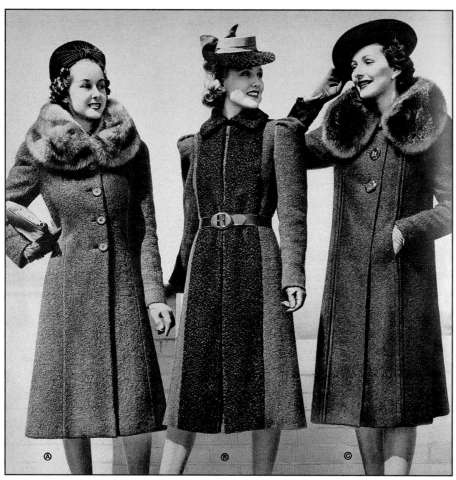

Boucle coats, warmly interlined, to keep the cold away. *Fall/Winter 1939-1940*

For the woman who wants to look slimmer, these coats are trim and sleek. *Fall/Winter 1939-1940*

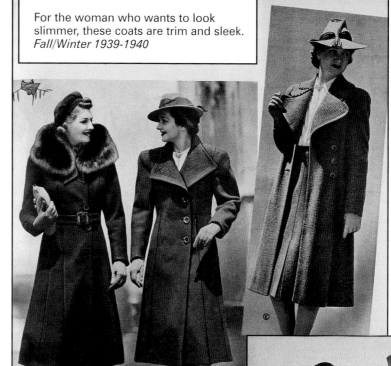

2-piece man tailored suits are newer, smarter, and more flattering than ever! Top it off with a classic Swagger coat that makes a woman look her feminine best. *Fall/Winter 1939-1940*

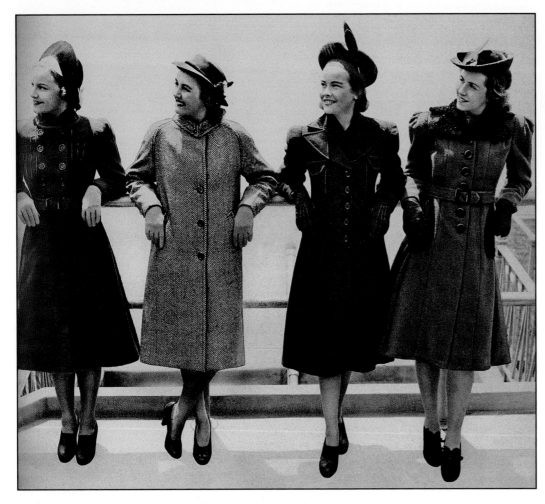

Swing Skirt Sports coat, Collegiate reversible is water repellent, The Reefer with dressmaker tucks, and the popular Princess with fur fabric collar. All styles that stand out. *Fall/Winter 1939-1940*

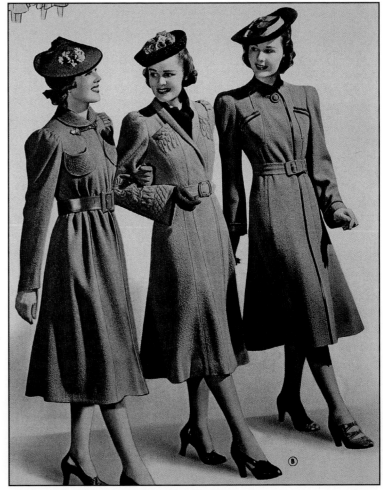

The new Angel Silhouette coat is fashion news, can be worn with or without the belt for two different looks, has squarish padded shoulders, high crescent stitched pockets with a Rayon hankie, in All Wool Crepe with Rayon Faille lining. Trapunto coat has quilted embroidery on sleeves and pockets, a full gored flaring skirt with beautiful seaming, of All Wool Crepe with Silk Crepe lining and comes with a harmonizing Rayon Crepe scarf. Velvet Bound Cardigan coat is an All Wool Crepe lined with Silk Crepe, has wide sleeves, double triangular pockets, and rich Rayon Velvet bindings. *Spring/Summer 1939*

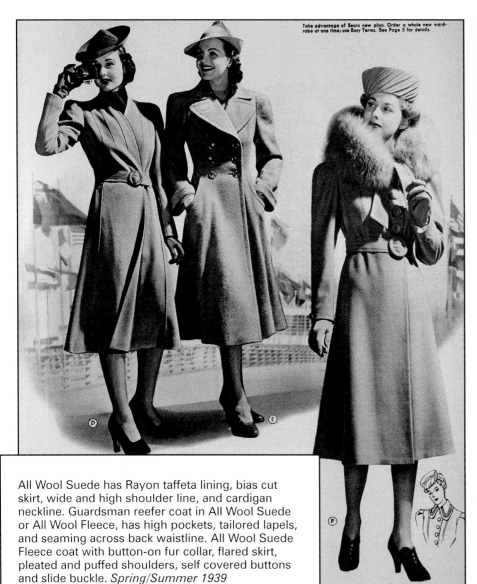

All Wool Suede has Rayon taffeta lining, bias cut skirt, wide and high shoulder line, and cardigan neckline. Guardsman reefer coat in All Wool Suede or All Wool Fleece, has high pockets, tailored lapels, and seaming across back waistline. All Wool Suede Fleece coat with button-on fur collar, flared skirt, pleated and puffed shoulders, self covered buttons and slide buckle. *Spring/Summer 1939*

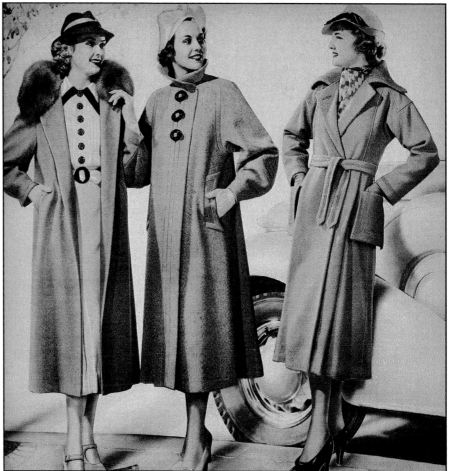

Dashalaine Polo coats are made of All-Wool, lined with All Rayon Earl-Glo. Rich, fleecy-soft, and luxurious. *Spring/Summer 1937*

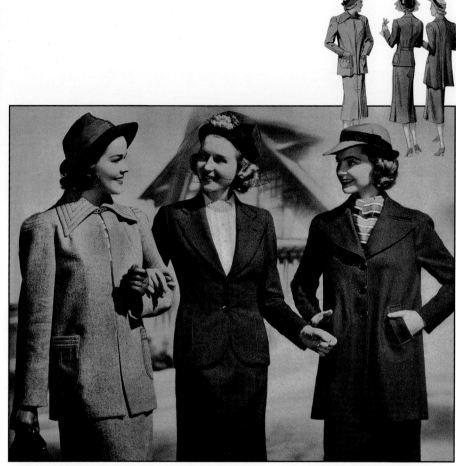

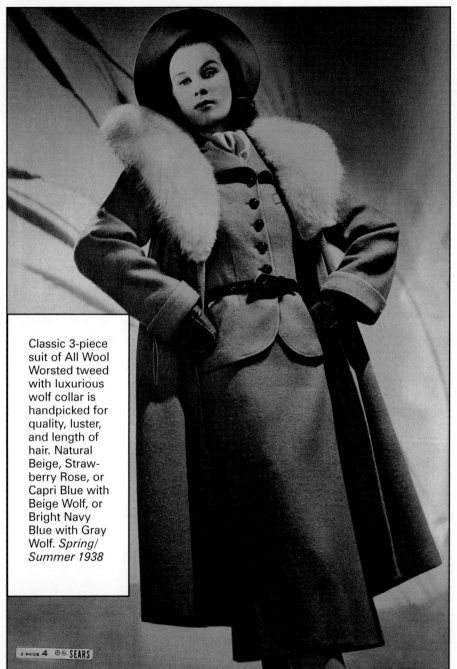

Classic 3-piece suit of All Wool Worsted tweed with luxurious wolf collar is handpicked for quality, luster, and length of hair. Natural Beige, Strawberry Rose, or Capri Blue with Beige Wolf, or Bright Navy Blue with Gray Wolf. *Spring/ Summer 1938*

Dressy swagger suit in rich All Wool has broad stitched shoulders, trim young collar with a metal chain fastener, unlined jacket, and novelty pockets in Copen Blue, Melon Rust, Light Fog Gray, and Medium Tan. Men's-Wear type suit with jacket lined in rayon taffeta, kick-pleated shirt, in Navy Blue, Medium Gray, and Medium Brown. Topper suit in All Wool has an unlined coat and skirt with side pleats and wide hem in Copen Blue, Strawberry Rose, and Navy Blue. *Spring/ Summer 1938*

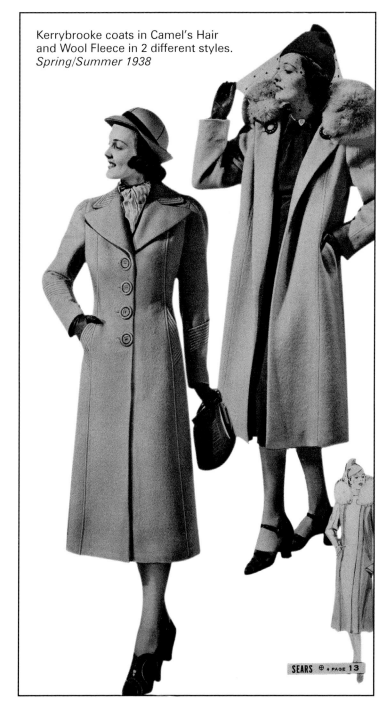

Kerrybrooke coats in Camel's Hair and Wool Fleece in 2 different styles.
Spring/Summer 1938

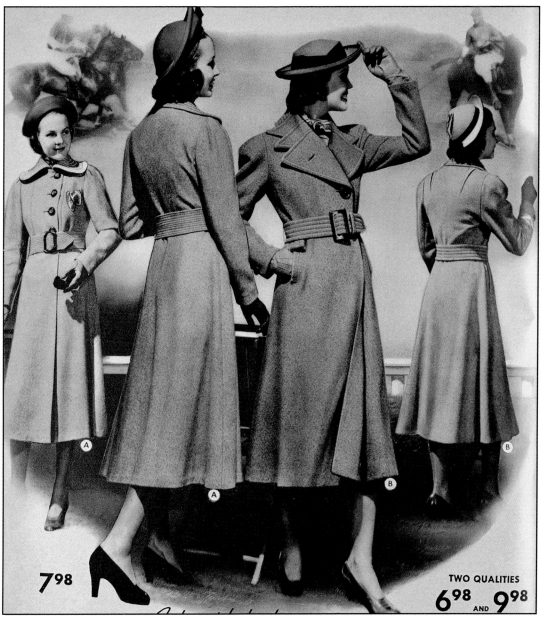

7⁹⁸

TWO QUALITIES
6⁹⁸ AND 9⁹⁸

Polo coats in wool/rayon and wool. Sporty, smart, and very fashionable this spring.
Spring/Summer 1938

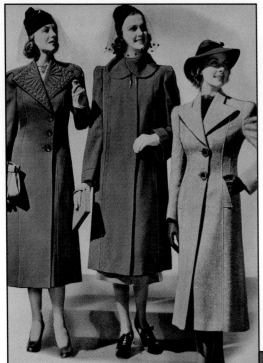

Trapunto stitching on All Wool Crepe with flattering Princess lines. Boxy Silhouette is the newest coat of the season with wide shoulders and straight full lines. Cereal Tweed in sleek fitted lines is suitable for sporty to dressy looks. *Spring/Summer 1938*

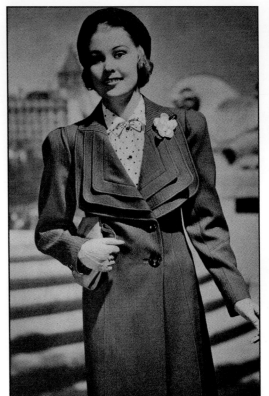

All Wool Crepe and All Wool Fleece give a slenderizing look to regular and stout sizes. *Spring/Summer 1938*

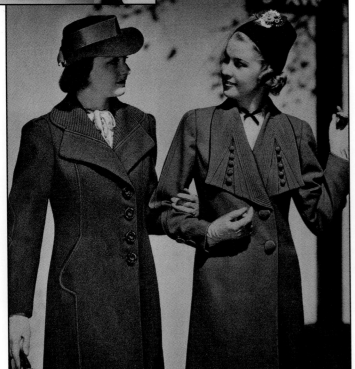

All Wool Shetland is beautifully stitched, superbly tailored, with expensive looking buttons. All Wool Worsted coat has very flattering collar, and weighted Silk Crepe lining. Both coats come in regular and shorter lengths. *Spring/Summer 1938*

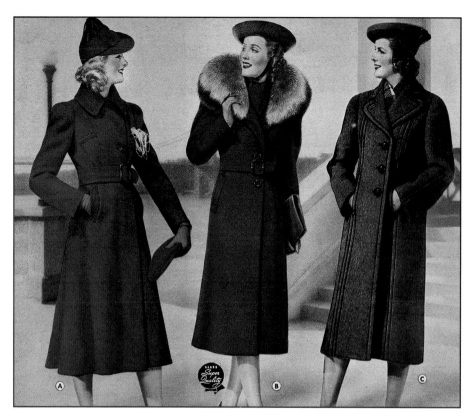

Quality Kerrybrooke coats in warm all wool suede fleece, all wool fleece with genuine raccoon fur, and fleece Swagger. *Fall/Winter 1938/1939*

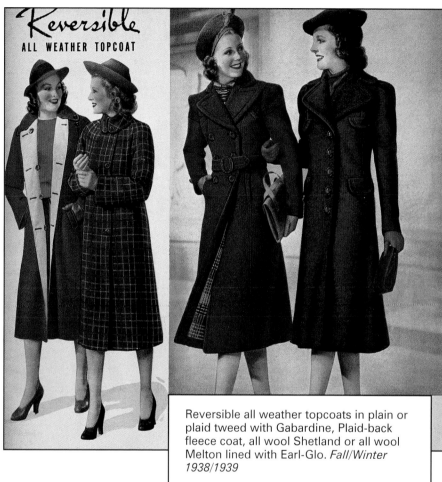

Reversible all weather topcoats in plain or plaid tweed with Gabardine, Plaid-back fleece coat, all wool Shetland or all wool Melton lined with Earl-Glo. *Fall/Winter 1938/1939*

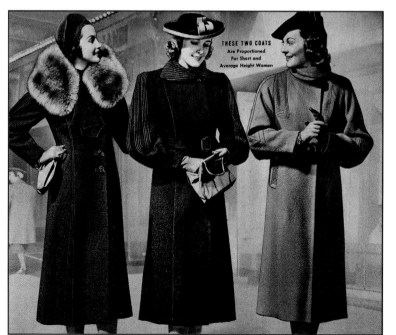

Charmodes are designed with youth in every line, a detachable fur collar on all wool, all wool crepe with Earl-Glo rayon satin, all wool fleece Swagger is smooth, soft, and marvelously warm. *Fall/Winter 1938/1939*

Rich all wool suiting has a luxurious fur collar on pleated swagger coat and a kick pleated skirt. All wool 3-piece suit has a contrasting knitted blouse, chic button jacket, and gored zip-placket skirt. Topcoat, jacket, and skirt in soft luscious Shetland. *Fall/Winter 1938/1939*

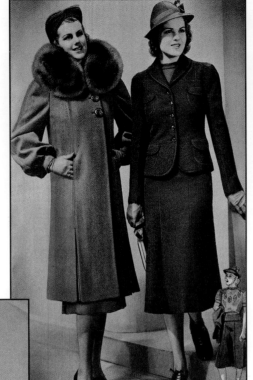

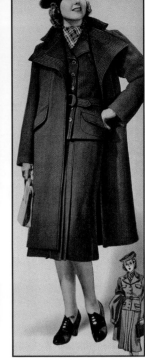

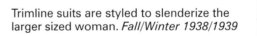

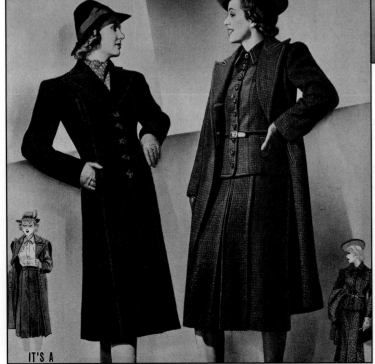

Trimline suits are styled to slenderize the larger sized woman. *Fall/Winter 1938/1939*

2-piece Reefer suit in all wool Shetland is flawlessly tailored with simple classic lines that will never go out of style. 3-piece suit in Checked suiting or all wool nubbed suiting. No wardrobe is complete without one. *Fall/Winter 1938/1939*

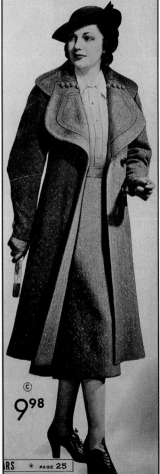

9⁹⁸

RS ✳ PAGE 25

IT'S A

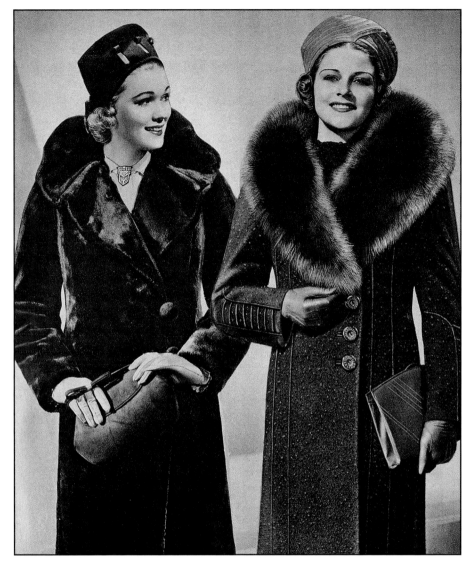

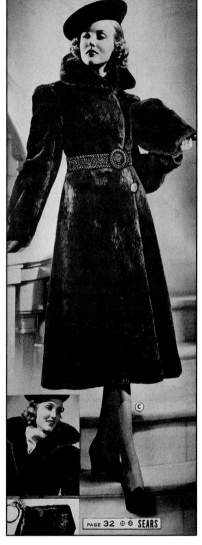

Princess flared genuine selected Coney fur coat, full cut swagger in Caracul Lamb fur or Moire Kid Caracul, and Trotteur Swagger in fine quality dyed Coney fur or "Empress Quality" dyed Coney. *Fall/Winter 1938/1939*

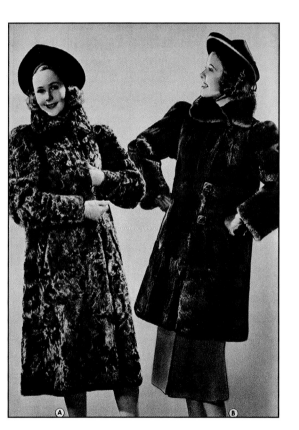

Trimline lustrous silk pile plush coat in black with a long collar that can be worn up or down. Bouclé Crepe coat with genuine Manchurian Wolf-dyed Dog Fur or Black-dyed Raccoon fur. *Fall/Winter 1938/1939*

Three color-correct and fashion-perfect costumes that can be worn to make you thrillingly young! *Fall/Winter 1937-1938*

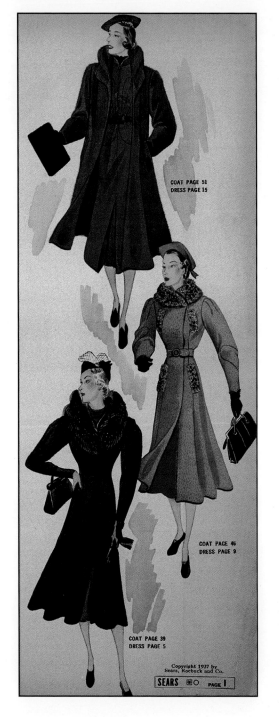

Furred swagger has tailor stitched gores to give that swing back look, tapered sleeves, in a quality fleece that is 70% wool. The new 1938 Silhouette has a flaring bias-cut skirt, stitched collar, wide stitched belt, and is half wool and balance rayon. *Fall/ Winter 1937-1938*

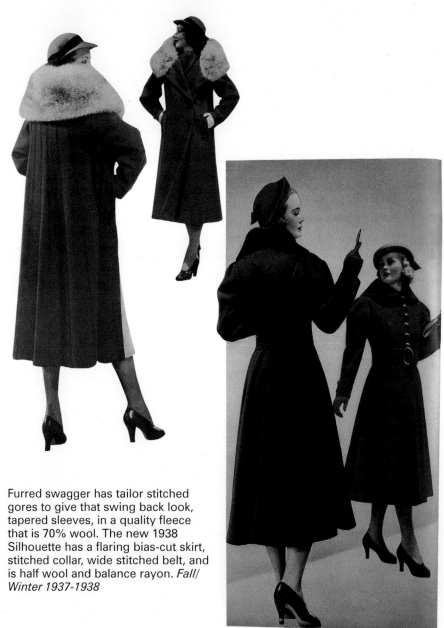

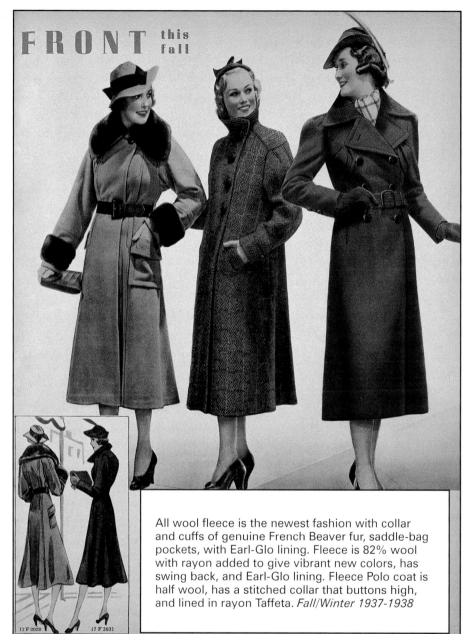

FRONT this fall

All wool fleece is the newest fashion with collar and cuffs of genuine French Beaver fur, saddle-bag pockets, with Earl-Glo lining. Fleece is 82% wool with rayon added to give vibrant new colors, has swing back, and Earl-Glo lining. Fleece Polo coat is half wool, has a stitched collar that buttons high, and lined in rayon Taffeta. *Fall/Winter 1937-1938*

17 F 2020   17 F 2031

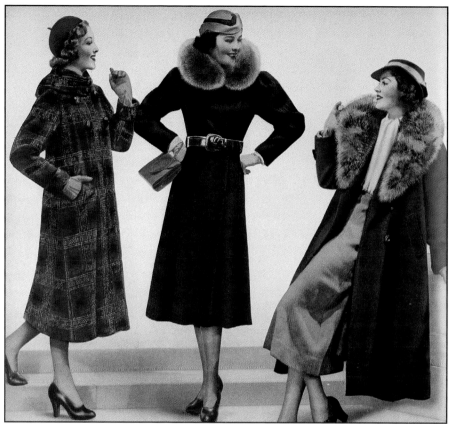

Kerrybrooke coats in sporty styles. Swagger coat has a hood and collar all in one, raglan sleeves, in wool and rayon. Warm fleece silhouette has a collar of genuine Manchurian wolf dyed dog fur, high placed pockets, and full gored skirt. with wide belt. Swagger with fluffy opossum fur collar, slot-seamed back and deep roomy pockets. *Fall/Winter 1937-1938*

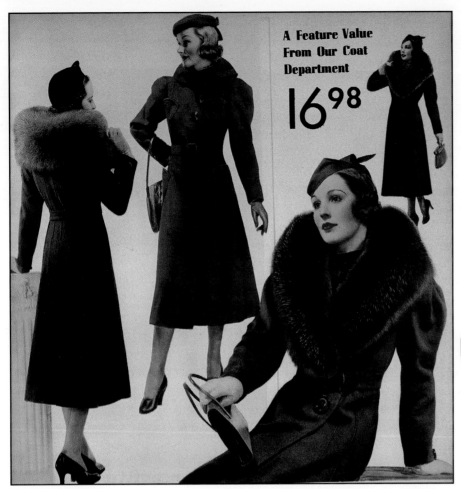

Novelty crepe coating has genuine Ibex fur, ten gores in the skirt, and Earl-Glo lining. All wool fleece has smart clinched-in waistline, wide shoulders, and flared skirt. Novelty crepe coating has Black Manchurian wolf dyed dog fur and is smartly designed to give you long, slim, flattering lines. *Fall/Winter 1937-1938*

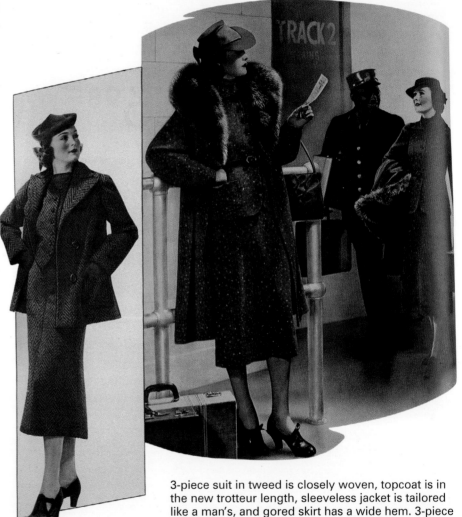

3-piece suit in tweed is closely woven, topcoat is in the new trotteur length, sleeveless jacket is tailored like a man's, and gored skirt has a wide hem. 3-piece tweed suit has magnificent raccoon collar on the topcoat, jacket is lined with satin and has a leather belt, and skirt has side kick pleats and a wide hem. *Fall/Winter 1937-1938*

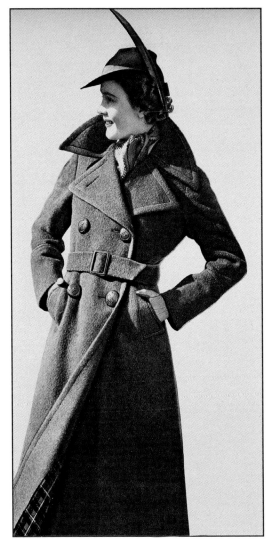

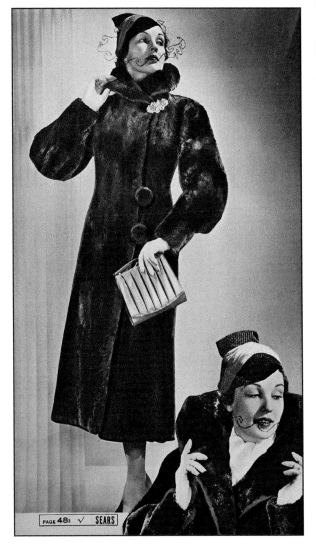

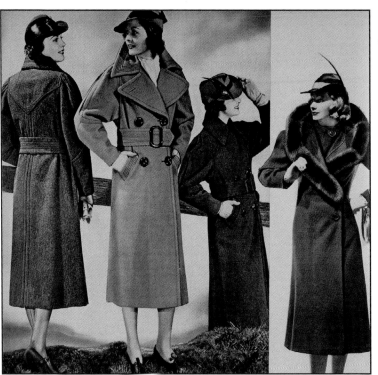

Miss America Polo coats with smart checks in heavy fleece, all wool shaggy fleece, and rich quality fleece. *Fall/Winter 1937-1938*

Polo coat is full-cut, has broad shoulders, deep pockets, and expensive looking big buttons. The felt hat is sponsored by a world famous designer, the side-rolled brim is turned down, and has a handsome feather. *Fall/Winter 1937-1938*

Northern Seal Dyed Coney or Beaver Dyed Coney coat with exquisite flower-petal collar fastens with a big rhinestone clip, has slender semi-fitted style, pleated runching at neck and wrists lessens wear on the fur, and lined in Duchess Satin. *Fall/Winter 1937-1938*

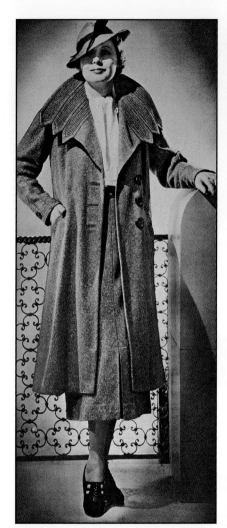

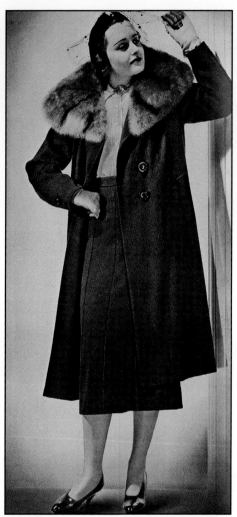

2-piece tweed suit has 46" swagger coat with the new lavishly stitched triple collar.
Slim lined skirt has front kick pleat and wide hem. 2-piece suit coat has a 2-way
collar in long-haired Fox-dyed Vicuna fur on heavy crepe coating, The tailored skirt
is trim and has a wide hem. *Fall/Winter 1937-1938*

Carefree stockings with Aqua-Sec beauty
treatment keeps them lovely to resist snags,
runs and rain spots. Clear, flawless, and
Ringfree! *Fall/Winter 1937-1938*

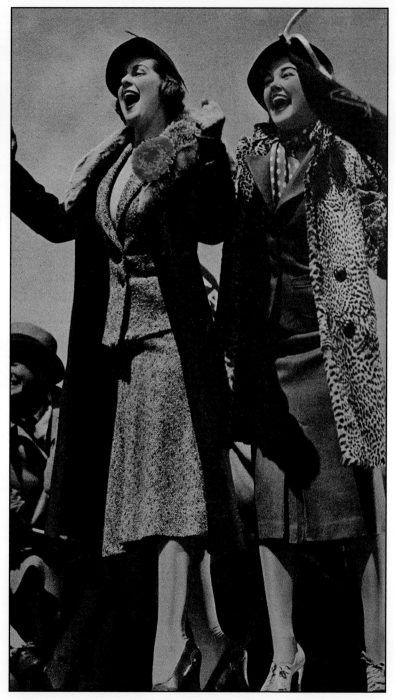

Rainwear

Pilofilm is the wonderful material developed from pure rubber that is transparent, featherlite, waterproof, and odorless. These raincoats and Visi-Brellas are made from this exciting new material. *Fall/Winter 1938/1939*

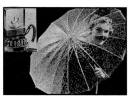

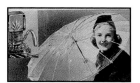

Visi-Brella's are made of sparkling pilofilm and offer safety in traffic. Raincoats and umbrellas to match are made of Rain-Bo-Film oiled silks. *Fall/Winter 1937-1938*

Accessories

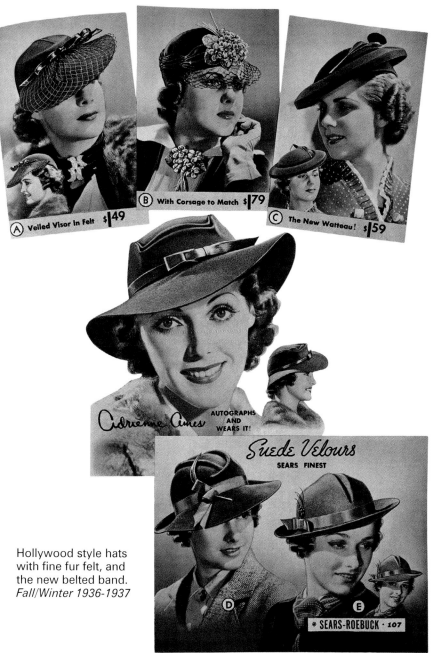

Hollywood style hats with fine fur felt, and the new belted band. *Fall/Winter 1936-1937*

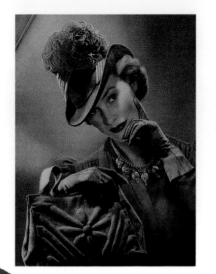

Accessories in Wintergreen are a sharp contrast to shades of brown, rust, and black. American Beauty is ideal paired with all blue and black colors. *Fall/Winter 1939-1940*

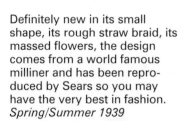

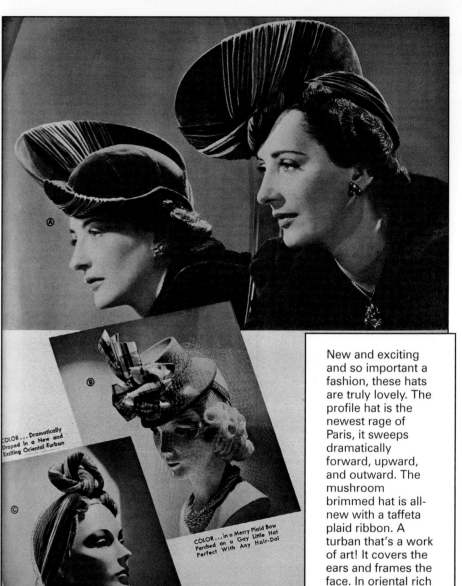

(A)

(B)

COLOR... Dramatically Draped in a New and Exciting Oriental Turban

(C)

COLOR... in a Merry Plaid Bow Perched on a Gay Little Hat Perfect With Any Hair-Do!

New and exciting and so important a fashion, these hats are truly lovely. The profile hat is the newest rage of Paris, it sweeps dramatically forward, upward, and outward. The mushroom brimmed hat is all-new with a taffeta plaid ribbon. A turban that's a work of art! It covers the ears and frames the face. In oriental rich colors, suede-like bagheera material. *Fall/Winter 1939-1940*

Definitely new in its small shape, its rough straw braid, its massed flowers, the design comes from a world famous milliner and has been reproduced by Sears so you may have the very best in fashion. *Spring/Summer 1939*

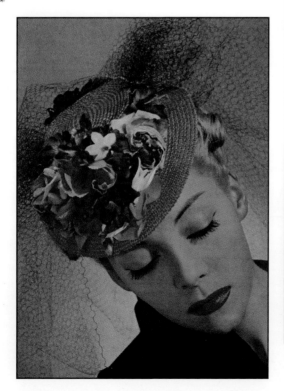

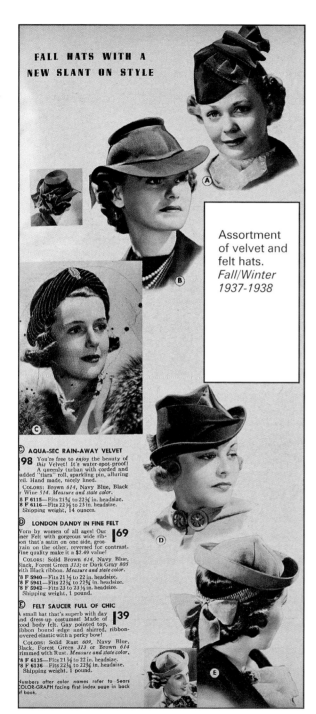

FALL HATS WITH A NEW SLANT ON STYLE

Assortment of velvet and felt hats. *Fall/Winter 1937-1938*

C AQUA-SEC RAIN-AWAY VELVET
98 You're free to *enjoy* the beauty of *this* Velvet! It's water-spot-proof! A queenly turban with corded and added "tiara" roll, sparkling pin, alluring veil. Hand made, nicely lined.
COLORS: Brown 614, Navy Blue, Black or Wine 514. *Measure and state color.*
8 F 6115—Fits 21¾ to 22¼ in. headsize.
8 F 6116—Fits 22½ to 23 in. headsize.
Shipping weight, 14 ounces.

D LONDON DANDY IN FINE FELT
169 Worn by women of all ages! Our finer Felt with gorgeous wide ribbon that's satin on one side, grosgrain on the other, reversed for contrast. Fine quality make it a $2.49 value!
COLORS: Solid Brown 614, Navy Blue, Black, Forest Green 313; or Dark Gray 805 with Black ribbon. *Measure and state color.*
8 F 5940—Fits 21½ to 22 in. headsize.
8 F 5941—Fits 22½ to 22¾ in. headsize.
8 F 5942—Fits 23 to 23½ in. headsize.
Shipping weight, 1 pound.

E FELT SAUCER FULL OF CHIC
139 A small hat that's superb with day and dress-up costumes! Made of good body felt. Gay pointed top, ribbon bound edge and shirred, ribbon-covered elastic with a perky bow!
COLORS: Solid Rust 609, Navy Blue, Black, Forest Green 313 or Brown 614 trimmed with Rust. *Measure and state color.*
8 F 6135—Fits 21½ to 22 in. headsize.
8 F 6136—Fits 22½ to 22¾ in. headsize.
Shipping weight, 1 pound.

Numbers after color names refer to Sears COLOR-GRAPH facing first index page in back of book.

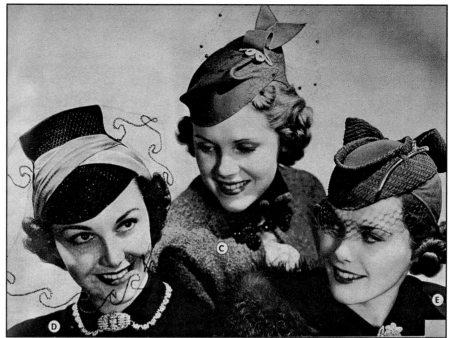

Turbans are high fashion for Fall with veils, bows, and ornaments. *Fall/ Winter 1937-1938*

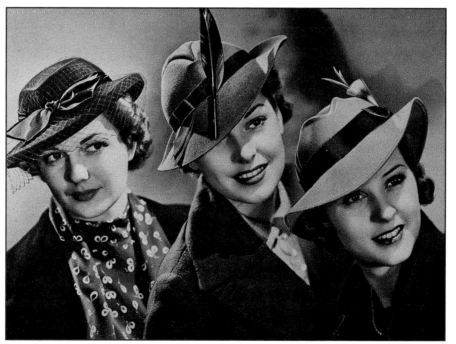

These hats are shaped to make your head look trim and smaller in bumper brim, and tucked crown styles. *Fall/Winter 1937-1938*

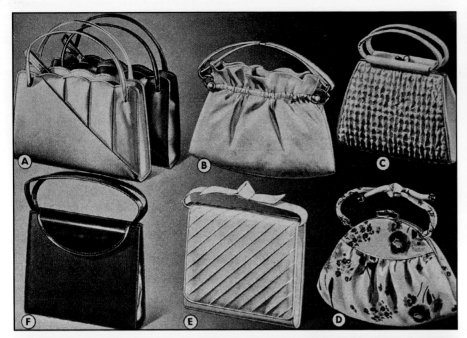

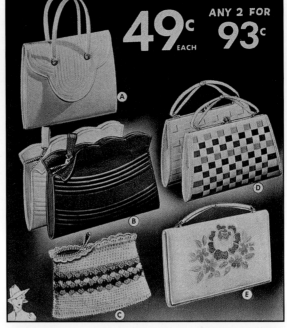

Handbags for all your outfits in artificial leathers, cottons, and celluloid's. *Spring/Summer 1938*

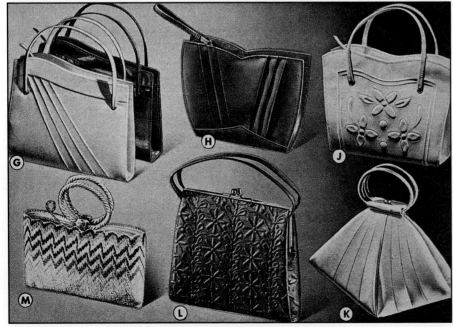

A selection of stylish handbags in fabrics such as artificial leather, crochet-effect rayon, and flowered prints. *Spring/Summer 1939*

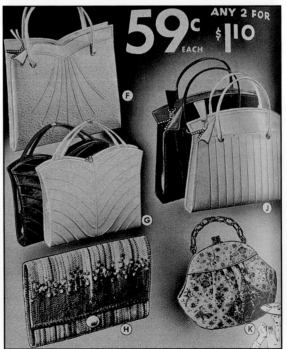

Shoes

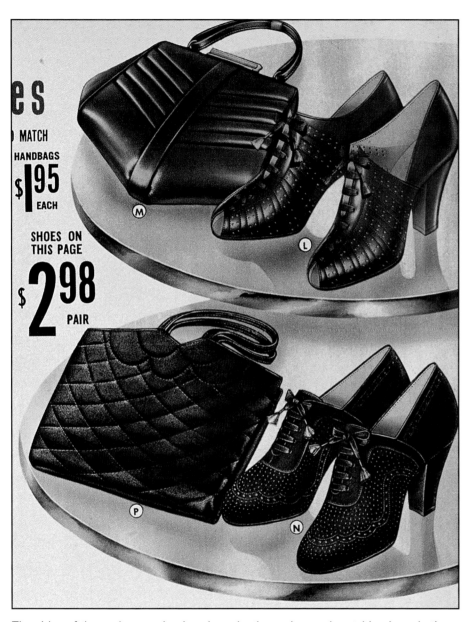

The sides of these shoes swing low, have leather soles, and matching bags in the finest styles. *Fall/Winter 1938/1939*

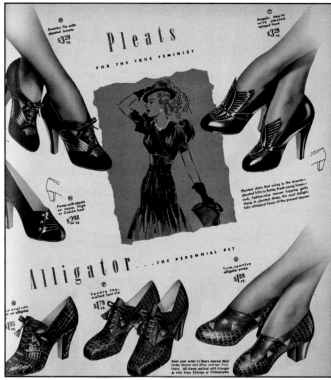

Leather pumps in high and low heels are the height of fashion. *Fall/Winter 1939-1940*

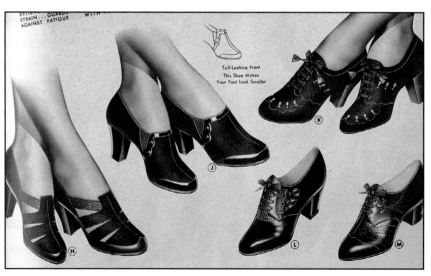

Women's shoes with a flared arch to relieve muscle strain, they are strong but lightweight for flexibility, and have a heel base of spongy rubber to take the jolts and jars out of walking. *Fall/Winter 1939-1940*

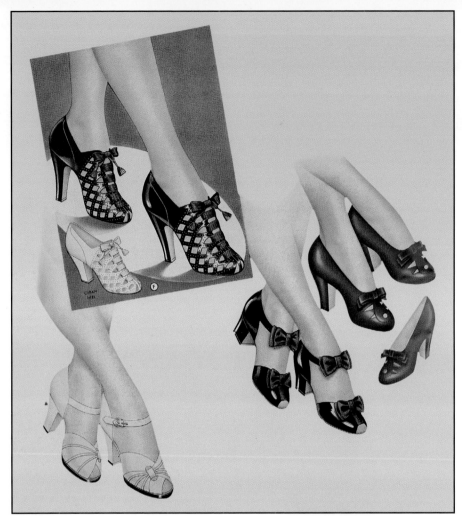

Foot flattery comes in large diamond-shaped cutouts all over the vamp with a Pussy Cat bow, Platform sandals with a peek at the toes, Doll shoes with two grosgrain ribbon bows, and a pump with cutouts and bow. *Spring/Summer 1939*

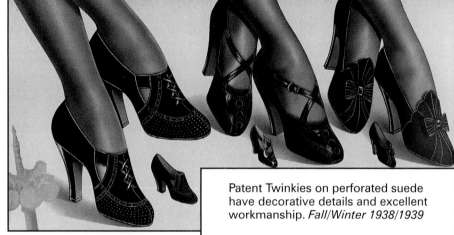

Patent Twinkies on perforated suede have decorative details and excellent workmanship. *Fall/Winter 1938/1939*

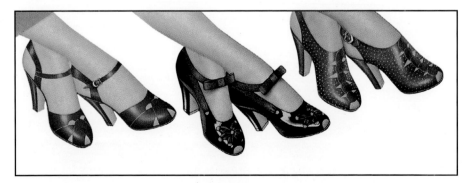

Shoes in select styles add color to your wardrobe. *Spring/Summer 1939*

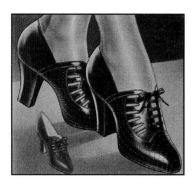
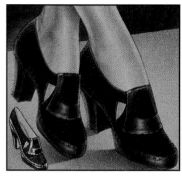
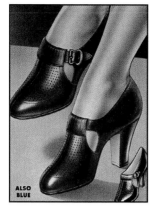
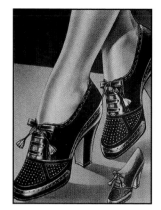

FOOTLINES come in a wide variety of styles to accessorize your wardrobe. *Fall/Winter 1938/1939*

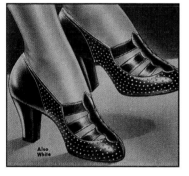
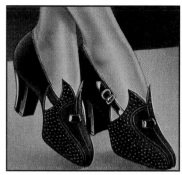
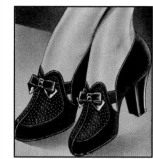
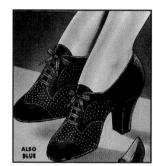

Young and old alike will find a style that's right for them in Flat-er-ease shoes. *Fall/ Winter 1938/1939*

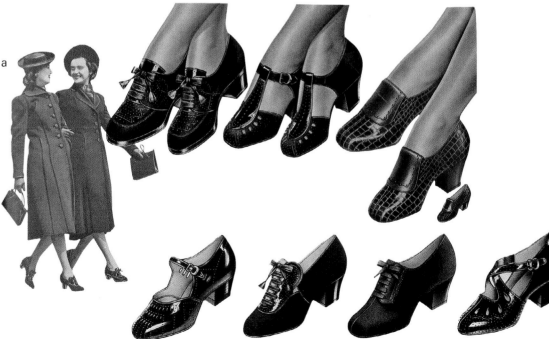

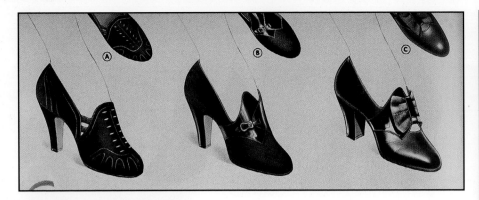

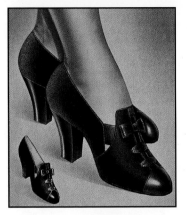

"Step-ins" flaunt new, up-in-front ideas. *Fall/Winter 1937-1938*

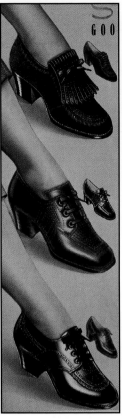

Soft suede with snap-on-tongue. Calfskin with rows of perforations, square toes, and rope stitching. Calfskin oxfords with moccasin style toe, and leather sole. All shoes are styled with Goodyear Welt durability. *Fall/Winter 1937-1938*

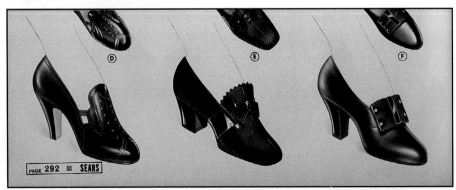

Styled with originality and good taste, priced for youthful budgets. *Fall/Winter 1937-1938*

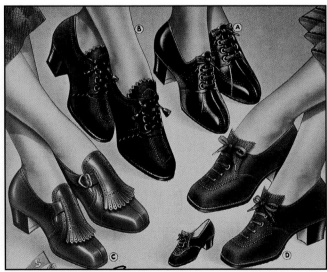

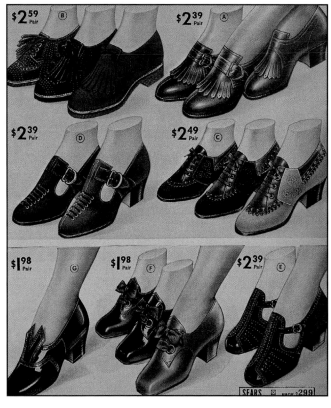

Young colorful fashions for mother and daughter. *Fall/Winter 1937-1938*

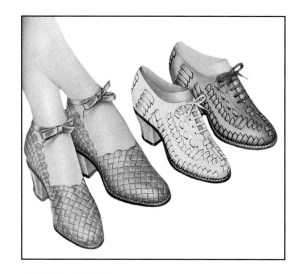

Huaraches are the newest in foot fashion. A peasant-style shoe that provides cool comfort. *Spring/Summer 1939*

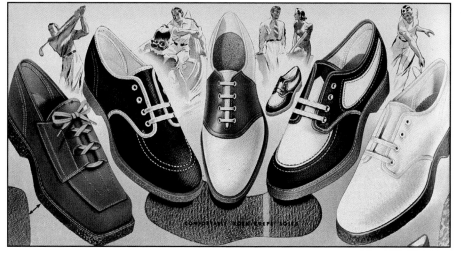

Fabric topped shoes for men and boys are the newest in summer footwear. Choose from "Box Car", Moccasin, "Saddles", Spectator, or Crepe Sole Sportsters styles. *Spring/Summer 1939*

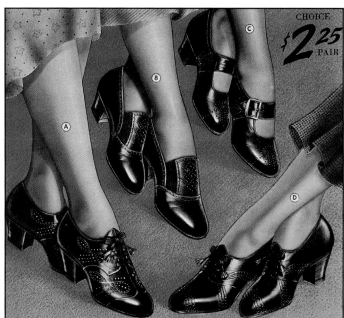

Famous Case shoes have free action support with built-in steel arch, no "breaking-in" flexible hand turned leather soles, in light and soft kidskin uppers that are so easy on the feet. *Fall/Winter 1937-1938*

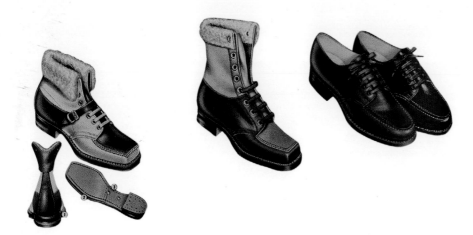

Snow boots for women are young and preppy and made for wintertime fun. Boots are cuffed to keep ankles warm and dry worn up or down. Moccasin shoes are soft, roomy, and strong. *Fall/Winter 1939-1940*

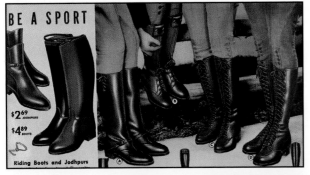

BE A SPORT

$2⁶⁹ JODHPURS

$4⁸⁹ BOOTS

Riding Boots and Jodhpurs

Step into style with a wide variety of boots from riding boots to jodhpurs, high or low cut boots, snow boots, and sports boots. *Fall/Winter 1938/1939*

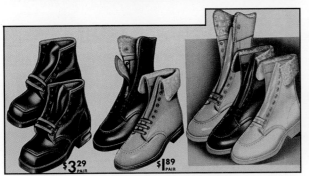

$3²⁹ PAIR

$1⁸⁹ PAIR

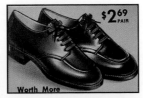

$2⁶⁹ PAIR

Worth More

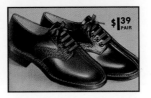

$1³⁹ PAIR

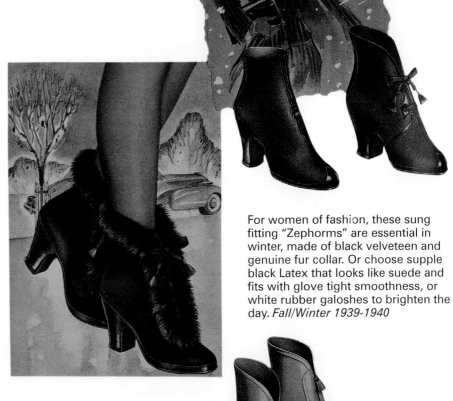

For women of fashion, these sung fitting "Zephorms" are essential in winter, made of black velveteen and genuine fur collar. Or choose supple black Latex that looks like suede and fits with glove tight smoothness, or white rubber galoshes to brighten the day. *Fall/Winter 1939-1940*

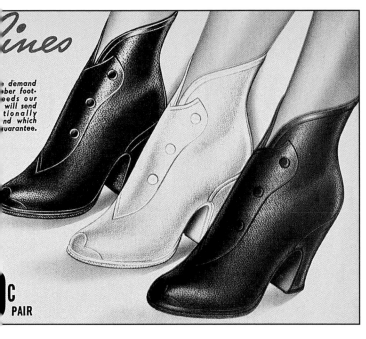

Trimlines are made of sturdy rubber, finished to look like fine kid, warm linings that slip on easily over suede or fabric shoes, and are light and smooth. *Fall/Winter 1938/1939*

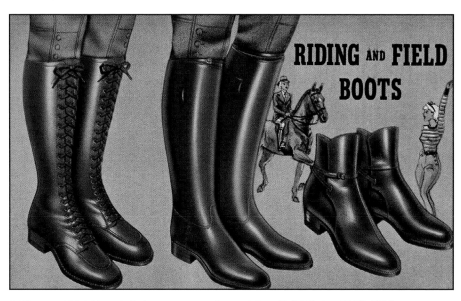

Riding and Field boots in lace-up or pull-on styles. *Fall/Winter 1937-1938*

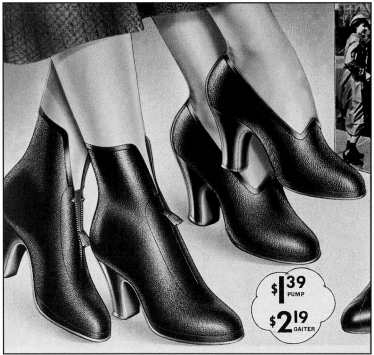

Rubber shoes and boots for cold or mild rainy days. *Fall/Winter 1937-1938*

"Zip" high cuts in hardy, smooth grain leather uppers with adjustable ankle lacings plus side fastener, stitch down leather sole, with low heel and rubber lift. *Fall/Winter 1937-1938*

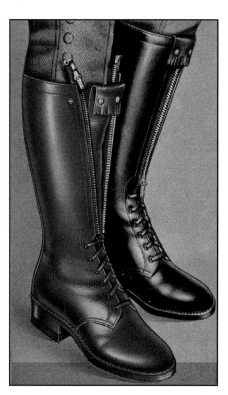

Teen Girls' Fashions

Dresses

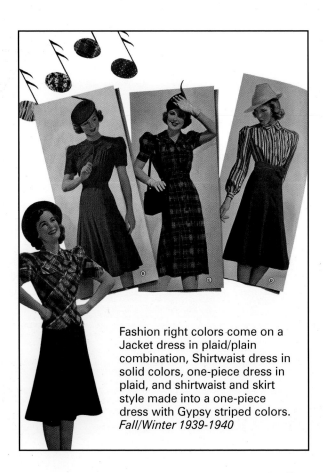

Fashion right colors come on a Jacket dress in plaid/plain combination, Shirtwaist dress in solid colors, one-piece dress in plaid, and shirtwaist and skirt style made into a one-piece dress with Gypsy striped colors. *Fall/Winter 1939-1940*

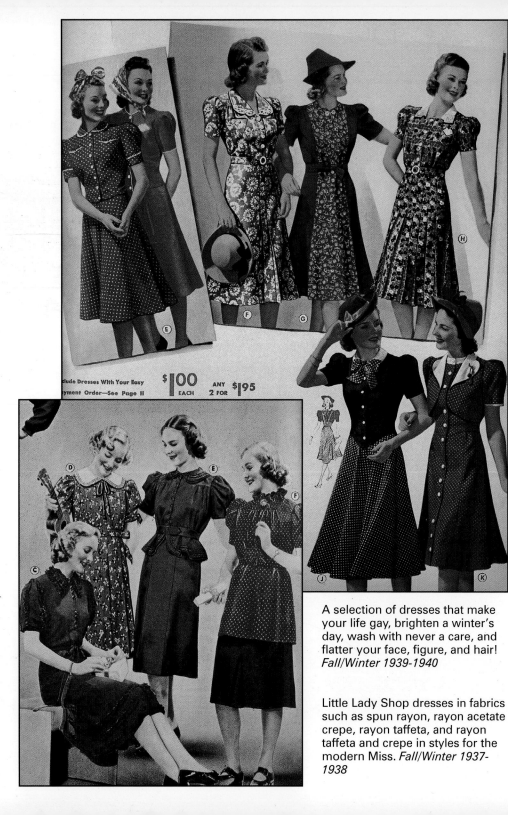

Include Dresses With Your Easy
Payment Order—See Page II
$**1**00 EACH ANY 2 FOR $**1**95

A selection of dresses that make your life gay, brighten a winter's day, wash with never a care, and flatter your face, figure, and hair! *Fall/Winter 1939-1940*

Little Lady Shop dresses in fabrics such as spun rayon, rayon acetate crepe, rayon taffeta, and rayon taffeta and crepe in styles for the modern Miss. *Fall/Winter 1937-1938*

Casual Separates

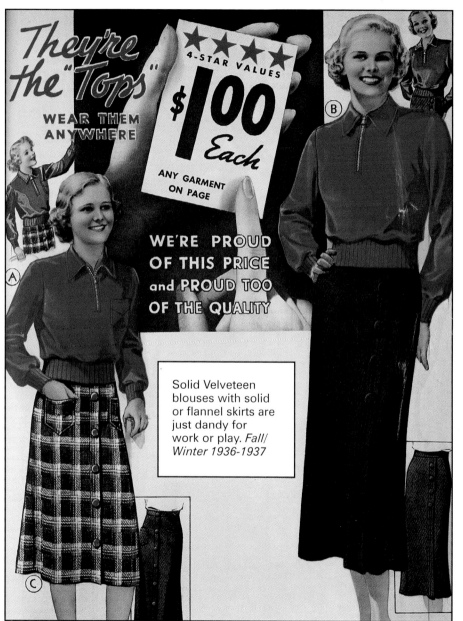

They're the "Tops"

WEAR THEM ANYWHERE

4-STAR VALUES

$100 Each

ANY GARMENT ON PAGE

WE'RE PROUD OF THIS PRICE and PROUD TOO OF THE QUALITY

Solid Velveteen blouses with solid or flannel skirts are just dandy for work or play. *Fall/ Winter 1936-1937*

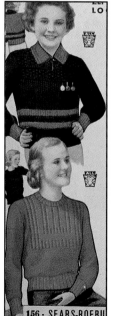

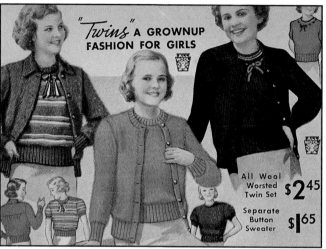

"Twins" A GROWNUP FASHION FOR GIRLS

All Wool Worsted Twin Set **$2⁴⁵**

Separate Button Sweater **$1⁶⁵**

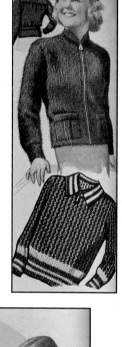

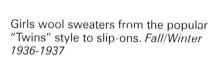

Girls wool sweaters from the popular "Twins" style to slip-ons. *Fall/Winter 1936-1937*

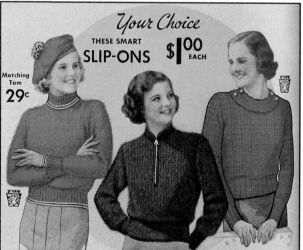

Your Choice

THESE SMART SLIP-ONS **$1⁰⁰ EACH**

Matching Tam 29c

156 · SEARS-ROEBU

95

Sleepwear

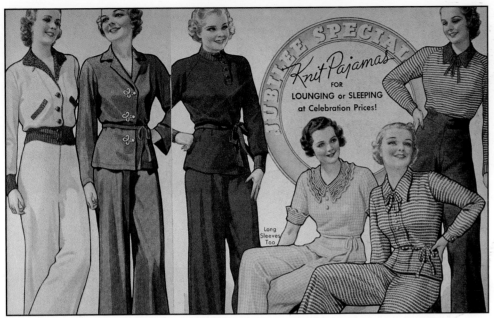

Comfortable and warm knit pajamas for lounging and sleeping, in solids or stripes.
Fall/Winter 1936-1937

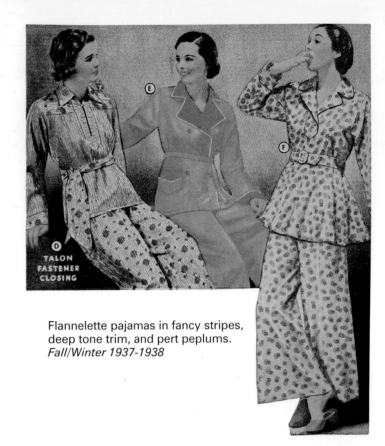

Flannelette pajamas in fancy stripes,
deep tone trim, and pert peplums.
Fall/Winter 1937-1938

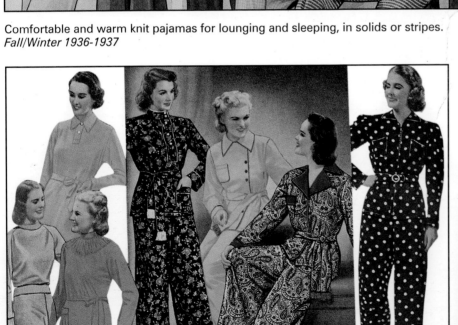

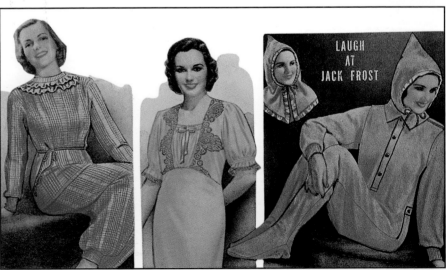

Pajamas, gowns, and sleepers in solids, polka dots, and prints. *Fall/Winter 1938/1939*

Sportswear

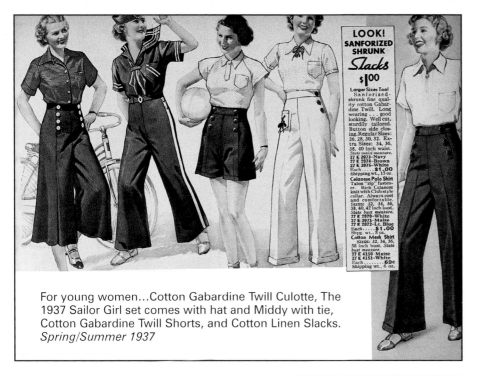

For young women…Cotton Gabardine Twill Culotte, The 1937 Sailor Girl set comes with hat and Middy with tie, Cotton Gabardine Twill Shorts, and Cotton Linen Slacks. *Spring/Summer 1937*

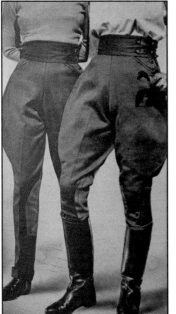

Jodhpurs and breeches have high waistbands to support the back and give trimmer waistlines. *Fall/Winter 1937-1938*

2-piece bike or tennis suit tailored in percale has a one piece play suit with short sleeve top, two-button front closing, and a patch pocket. When you need more femininity, slip on the wrap-around skirt that buttons all the way down the front. Beauty contest winner Eileen Drury wore this suit! *Spring/Summer 1938*

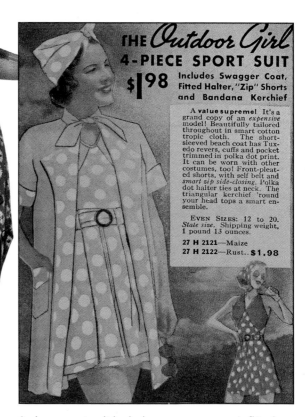

4-piece sport suit includes a swagger coat, fitted halter, zip shorts, and bandana kerchief. Tailored in cotton tropic cloth in a polka dot print. It is a grand copy of an *expensive* model! *Spring/Summer 1938*

Outerwear

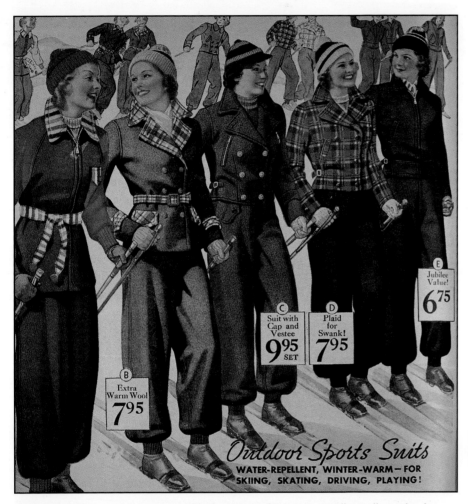

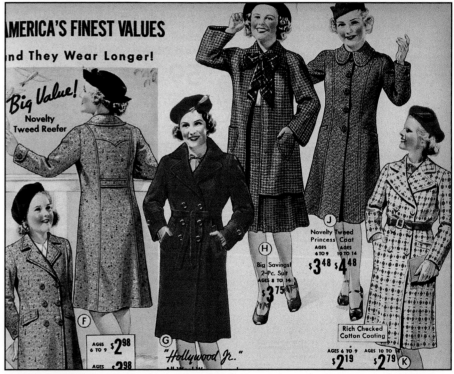

Dress warm for outdoor sports with these swanky water repellent all wool suits. Bottoms have solid colors, jackets have solid colors or solid/plaid combinations. *Fall/Winter 1936-1937*

An assortment of Classmate coats for girls in fabrics such All Wool and Cotton. *Spring/Summer 1937*

Kerrybrooke outdoor suits are water repellent and extra warm with cotton flannel lining in colors and styles to "suit" you. *Fall/Winter 1937-1938*

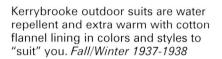

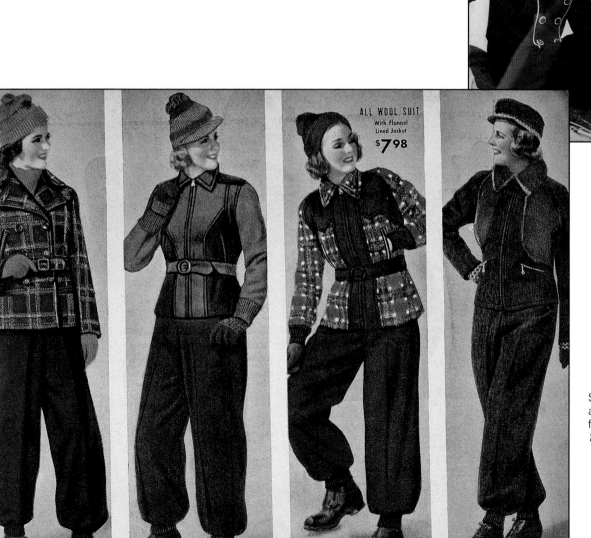

ALL WOOL SUIT
With Flannel
Lined Jacket
$7.98

Snowsuits of half wool, all wool, and Byrd cloth to keep you warm for outdoor winter fun. *Fall/Winter 1938/1939*

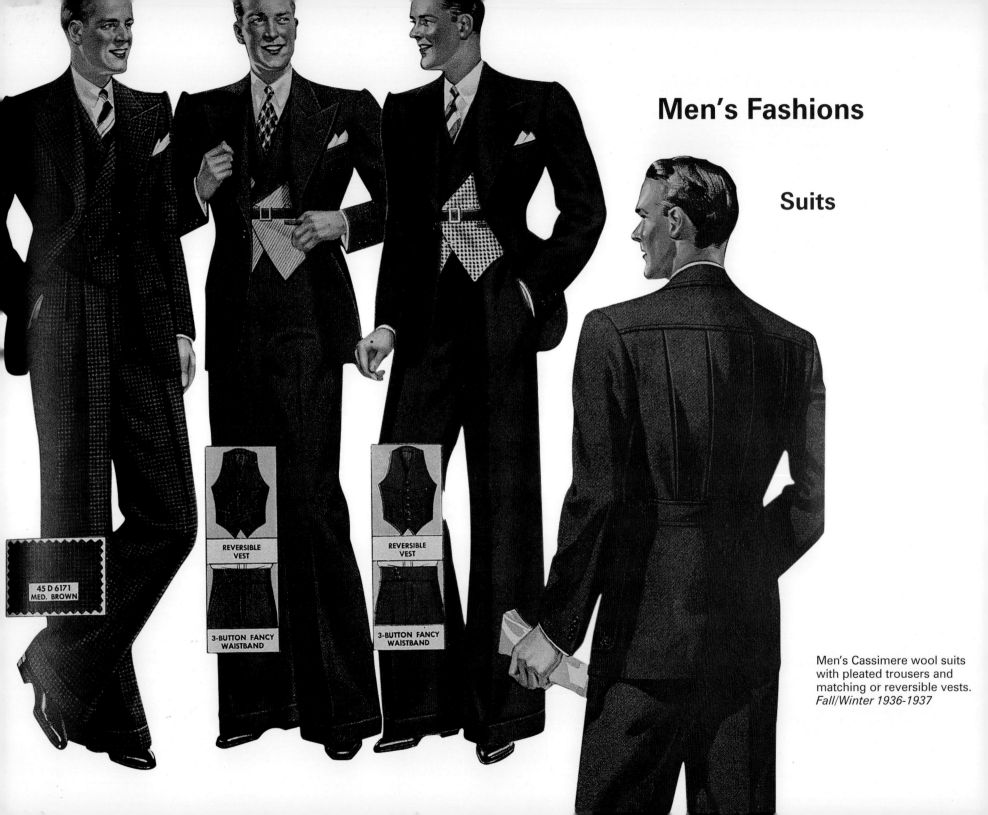

Men's Fashions

Suits

45 D 6171
MED. BROWN

REVERSIBLE
VEST

3-BUTTON FANCY
WAISTBAND

REVERSIBLE
VEST

3-BUTTON FANCY
WAISTBAND

Men's Cassimere wool suits
with pleated trousers and
matching or reversible vests.
Fall/Winter 1936-1937

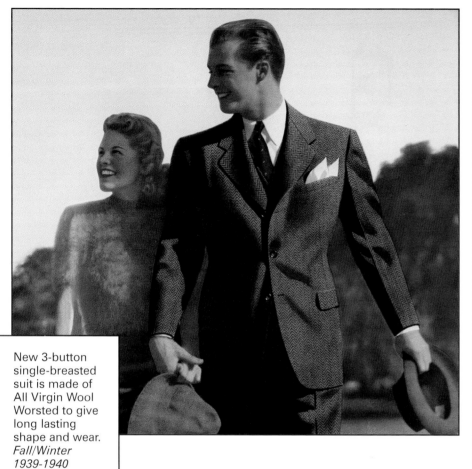

New 3-button single-breasted suit is made of All Virgin Wool Worsted to give long lasting shape and wear. *Fall/Winter 1939-1940*

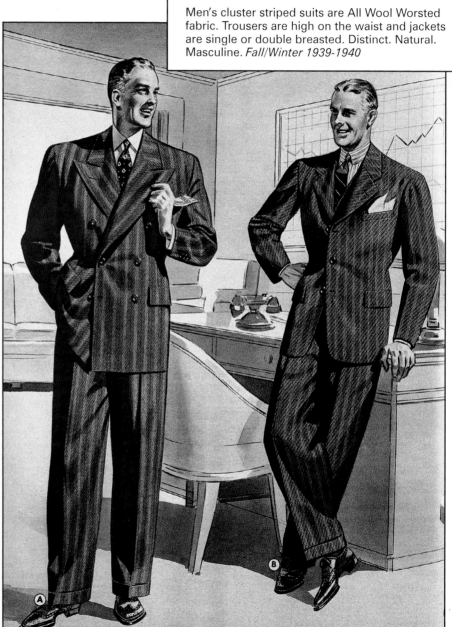

Men's cluster striped suits are All Wool Worsted fabric. Trousers are high on the waist and jackets are single or double breasted. Distinct. Natural. Masculine. *Fall/Winter 1939-1940*

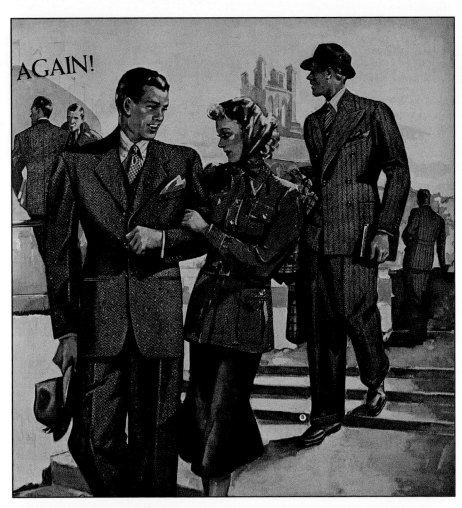

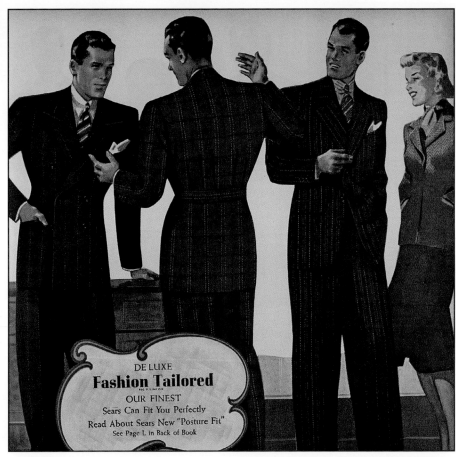

Tyrolean Tweed has All Wool Herringbone weave and is colorfully nubbed. It is a brand new California type semi-drape with gusseted shoulders, British high-rise trousers with full draping pleats in Brown or Green. Herringbone Worsted of smooth All Wool with popular stripes, dressy patch pocket, and is double breasted in Green or Blue. *Fall/Winter 1939-1940*

Sears finest fashion tailored suits in Clean-Cut, Sports Back, and Classic styles. *Fall/Winter 1939-1940*

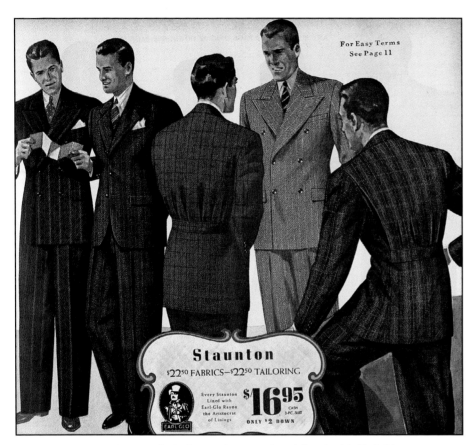

Staunton

$22⁵⁰ FABRICS—$22⁵⁰ TAILORING

Every Staunton
Lined with
Earl-Glo Rayon
the Aristocrat
of Linings

EARL GLO

$16⁹⁵
CASH
3-PC. SUIT

ONLY $2 DOWN

Men's Staunton suits are all virgin wool worsted and lined with Earl-Glo rayon. Striped double breasted, Broad Shoulder Drape, 2 Button Sunburst Sports Back, Chalk Stripes, and New Action Back styles are pictured. *Fall/Winter 1939-1940*

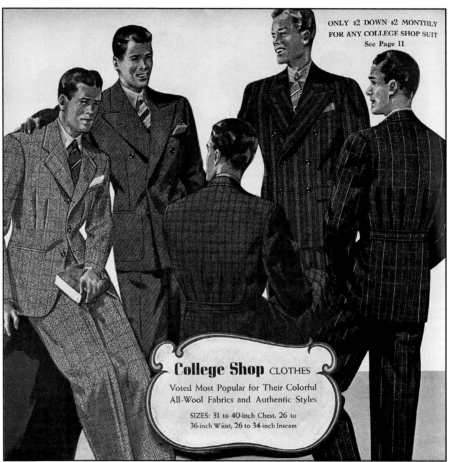

College Shop CLOTHES

Voted Most Popular for Their Colorful
All-Wool Fabrics and Authentic Styles

SIZES: 31 to 40-inch Chest, 26 to
36-inch Waist, 26 to 34-inch Inseam

All wool cassimere in a fancy striped herringbone pattern. Patch pocket double-breasted suit with sports back. All virgin wool worsted woven check pattern is double-breasted, has patch pockets, and 21" trouser cuffs. All Virgin wool worsted in cluster-stripe pattern with pleated trousers. Striped overplaid suit in all virgin wool worsted, has "Sunburst" sports back and patch pockets. *Fall/Winter 1939-1940*

High Style suits for men including the dashing swagger model with All Wool Cassimere, peak lapels, high cushion shoulders, double breasted reversible vest featuring a decorative buckle, and wide 22" cuff bottoms. All Wool Cassimere in checked pattern is all new for 1937 and has new Bi-swing action back, peak lapels, patch pockets, wide cushioned shoulders, double breasted vest, and snappy pleated trousers. 100% Virgin Wool Worsted in small check weave pattern is brilliantly styled, and is smoothly tailored. All Wool Cassimere is a very popular style with double breasted sports-back coat, windowpane check pattern, and pleated trousers. *Spring/Summer 1937*

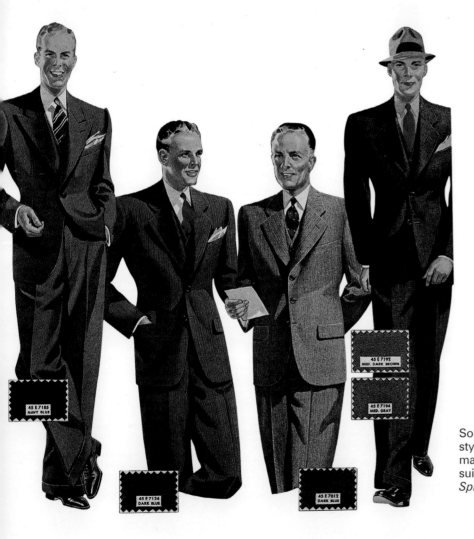

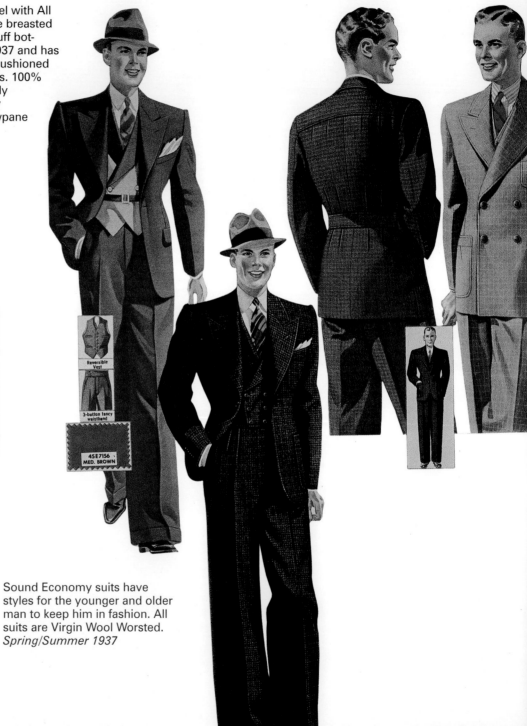

Reversible Vest

3-button fancy waistband

45 E 7156
MED. BROWN

45 E 7185
NAVY BLUE

45 E 7124
DARK BLUE

45 E 7012
DARK BLUE

45 E 7192
MED. DARK BROWN

45 E 7194
MED. GRAY

Sound Economy suits have styles for the younger and older man to keep him in fashion. All suits are Virgin Wool Worsted. *Spring/Summer 1937*

104

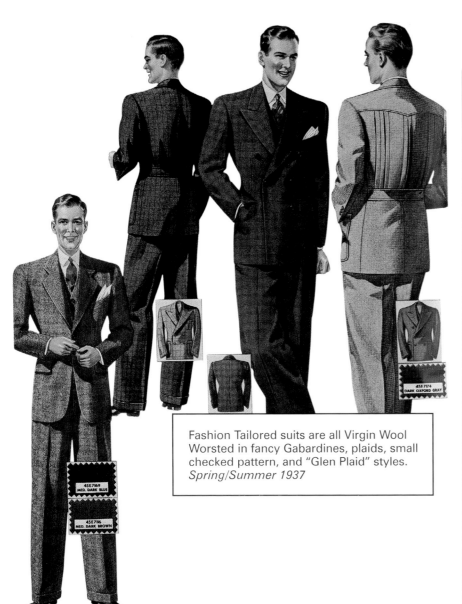

Fashion Tailored suits are all Virgin Wool Worsted in fancy Gabardines, plaids, small checked pattern, and "Glen Plaid" styles. *Spring/Summer 1937*

45E7169
MED. DARK BLUE

45E7116
MED. DARK BROWN

45E7174
DARK OXFORD GRAY

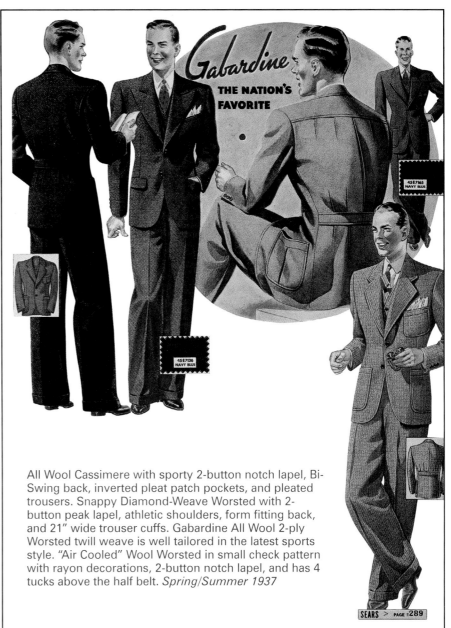

Gabardine

THE NATION'S FAVORITE

45E7165
NAVY BLUE

45E7136
NAVY BLUE

All Wool Cassimere with sporty 2-button notch lapel, Bi-Swing back, inverted pleat patch pockets, and pleated trousers. Snappy Diamond-Weave Worsted with 2-button peak lapel, athletic shoulders, form fitting back, and 21" wide trouser cuffs. Gabardine All Wool 2-ply Worsted twill weave is well tailored in the latest sports style. "Air Cooled" Wool Worsted in small check pattern with rayon decorations, 2-button notch lapel, and has 4 tucks above the half belt. *Spring/Summer 1937*

SEARS > PAGE 289

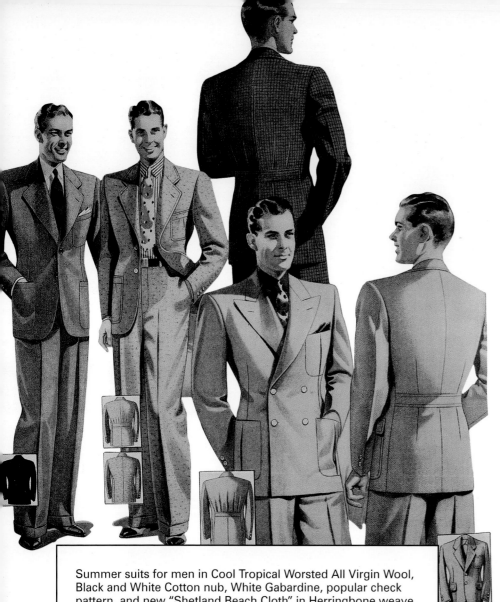

Summer suits for men in Cool Tropical Worsted All Virgin Wool, Black and White Cotton nub, White Gabardine, popular check pattern, and new "Shetland Beach Cloth" in Herringbone weave. *Spring/Summer 1937*

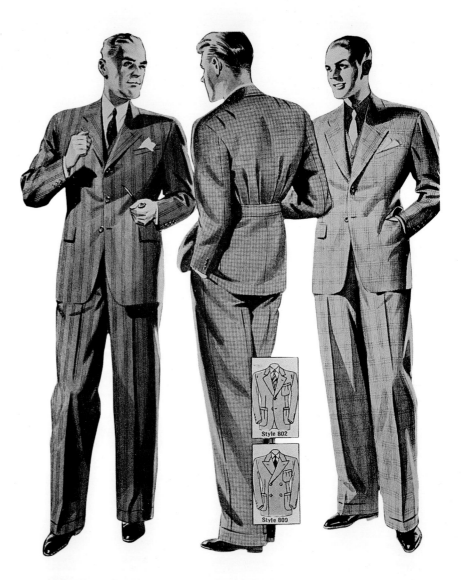

Style 802

Style 800

Made-To-Order men's suits lets you choose the fabric, style, and colors that you want. *Spring/Summer 1937*

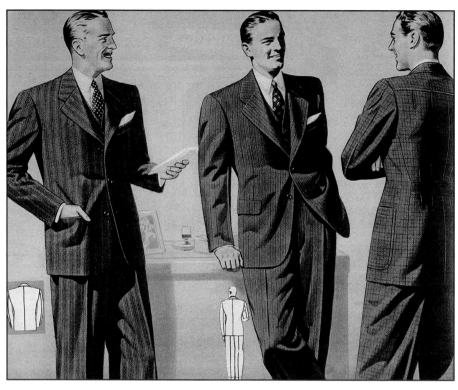

Smart and conservative all virgin wool suit is carefully tailored with genuine Hymo interlining. Single breasted pure virgin worsted suit with Earl-Glo rayon lining in a highly popular style. Double breasted suit of virgin wool worsted suit has patch pockets, sports back, and guaranteed to fit in every way. *Fall/Winter 1938/1939*

Staunton suits in the latest striped patterns, sports backs, single and double breasted, and overplaid designs. *Fall/Winter 1938/1939*

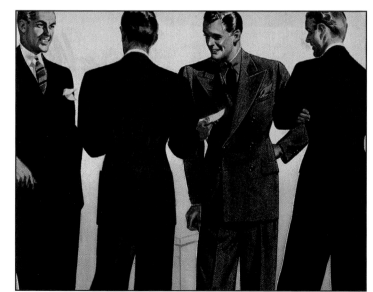

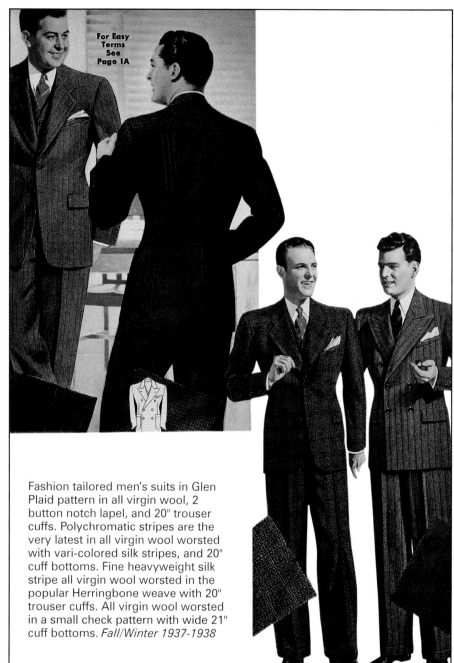

For Easy Terms See Page 1A

Fashion tailored men's suits in Glen Plaid pattern in all virgin wool, 2 button notch lapel, and 20" trouser cuffs. Polychromatic stripes are the very latest in all virgin wool worsted with vari-colored silk stripes, and 20" cuff bottoms. Fine heavyweight silk stripe all virgin wool worsted in the popular Herringbone weave with 20" trouser cuffs. All virgin wool worsted in a small check pattern with wide 21" cuff bottoms. *Fall/Winter 1937-1938*

107

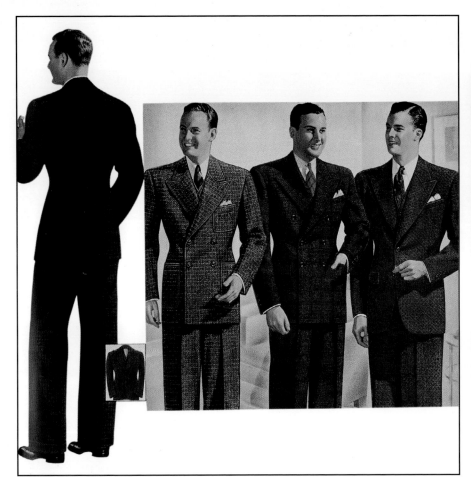

Small check weave pattern on all virgin wool worsted with tailored sports back, and 21" trouser cuffs. Windowpane check pattern all wool cassimere, double-breasted model with wide lapels, and 21" trouser cuffs. Worsted GlenPlaid with 3-button double-breasted coat with wide peak lapels, and 21" trouser cuffs. All virgin wool diamond weave, hard finished, pure Worsted with two-button peak lapel and 21" trouser cuffs. *Fall/Winter 1937-1938*

Workclothes

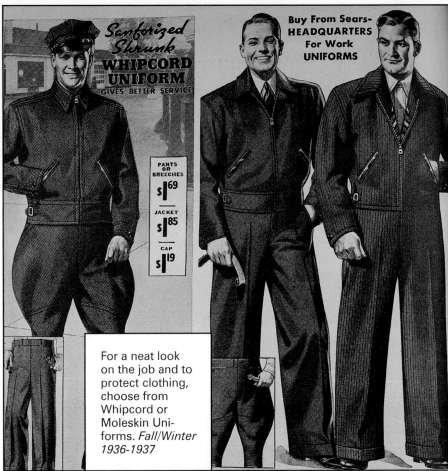

For a neat look on the job and to protect clothing, choose from Whipcord or Moleskin Uniforms. *Fall/Winter 1936-1937*

Sanforized-Shrunk work outfits are durable and strong enough for any job. *Spring/Summer 1938*

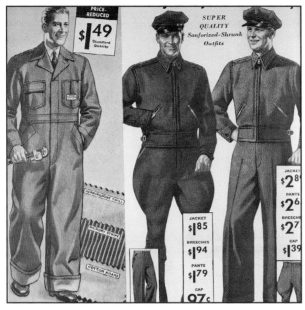

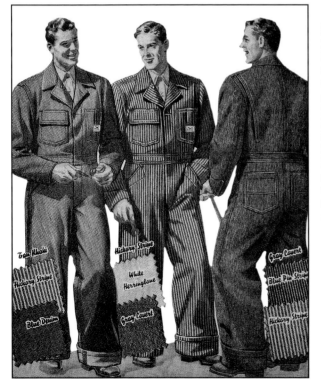

Hercules Nation-Alls are built for working comfort. Husky with button front are cut 6" larger than the chest size for extra room, and every main seam is triple stitched. Husky in Bi-Swing back is Sanforized-Shrunk, button-up front, and has big bellow pleats from shoulders to waist. Zip-front husky is Sanforized-Shrunk, has Bi-Swing back, and durable. *Fall/Winter 1939-1940*

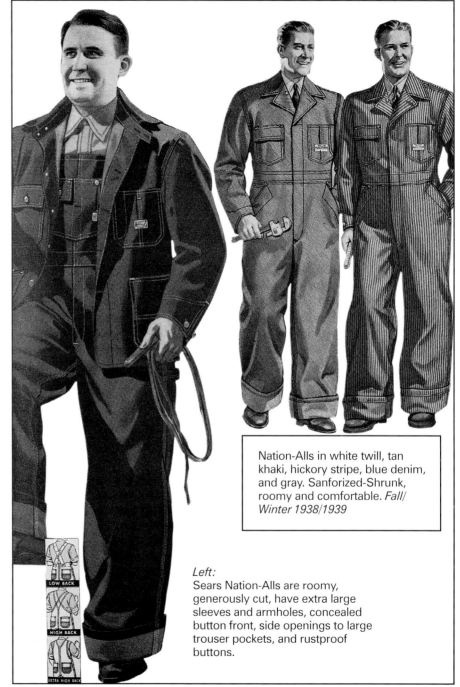

Nation-Alls in white twill, tan khaki, hickory stripe, blue denim, and gray. Sanforized-Shrunk, roomy and comfortable. *Fall/Winter 1938/1939*

Left:
Sears Nation-Alls are roomy, generously cut, have extra large sleeves and armholes, concealed button front, side openings to large trouser pockets, and rustproof buttons.

109

Drum Major overalls are of heavy white back drop tone indigo blue denim, Sanforized-Shrunk, cut extra large, double suspenders that will not curl or rust, two bib pockets, wide fly with 3 buttons, rip-proof triple stitched seams, strong hammer loop, rule pocket, and the jacket has four outside pockets with a double thickness at the bottom of the hip pockets. Both jacket and overalls are bartacked and reinforced at all strain points. Tough! *Spring/Summer 1937*

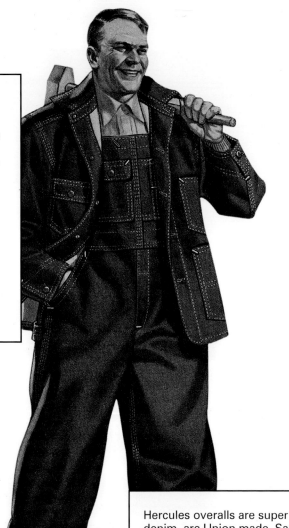

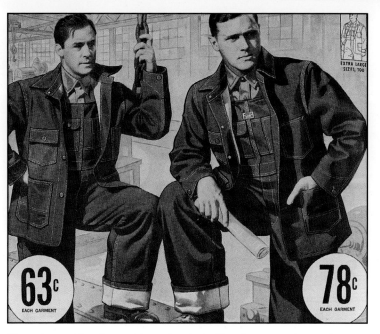

There is no skimping on these hard working heavy and extra heavy denim overalls. Triple stitched seams are rip proof, and all points of strain are reinforced and bar-tacked. *Fall/Winter 1938/1939*

Hercules overalls are super heavy, extra-strong denim, are Union made, Sanforized-shrunk, have triple stitched seams, and all pockets are self-faced which means there are no raw edges to curl and ravel. They are guaranteed to outwear any other overall, keep their color, and to hold their roomy fit. *Fall/Winter 1938/1939*

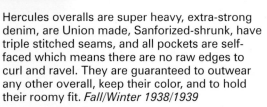

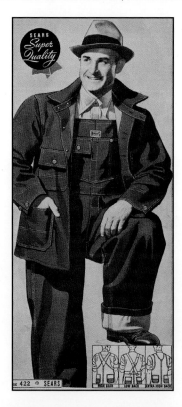

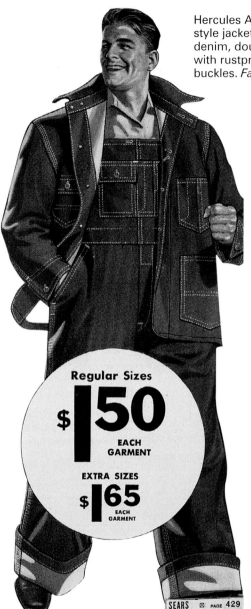

Hercules Apron style overalls and coat style jacket are extra heavy Blue Blood denim, double shrunk, triple stitched, with rustproof metal buttons and buckles. *Fall/Winter 1937-1938*

Regular Sizes
$ **150**
EACH GARMENT

EXTRA SIZES
$ **165**
EACH GARMENT

SEARS ⊠ PAGE 429

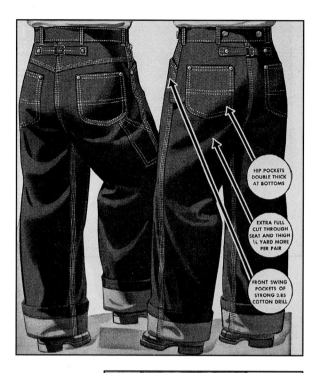

Denim work jeans are strong, extra heavy, and tough enough for any job. *Fall/Winter 1939-1940*

HIP POCKETS DOUBLE THICK AT BOTTOMS

EXTRA FULL CUT THROUGH SEAT AND THIGH ¼ YARD MORE PER PAIR

FRONT SWING POCKETS OF STRONG 2.85 COTTON DRILL

LOW BACK   HIGH BACK

Hercules Blue Blood Denim dunga-rees have extra heavy weight white back indigo blue denim, more threads to the inch, all pockets are double thick at the bottom, all seams triple-stitched, rustproof buttons, and adjustable back strap and buckle. Overalls to fit any man from short to tall and in between, in graduated patterns. *Fall/Winter 1937-1938*

Pacemaker, "Knee-Texed" overalls are an amazing improvement with extra heavy 8-ounce weight white back denim in indigo blue, Sanforized-Shrunk, double suspenders, two bib pockets reinforced with an extra strip of denim, boat sail drill front pockets, book, pencil and safety watch pocket, hammer loop, and guaranteed not to break buckles. *Spring/Summer 1937*

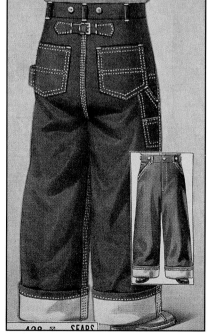

428 ⊠ SEARS

111

Casual and Sportswear

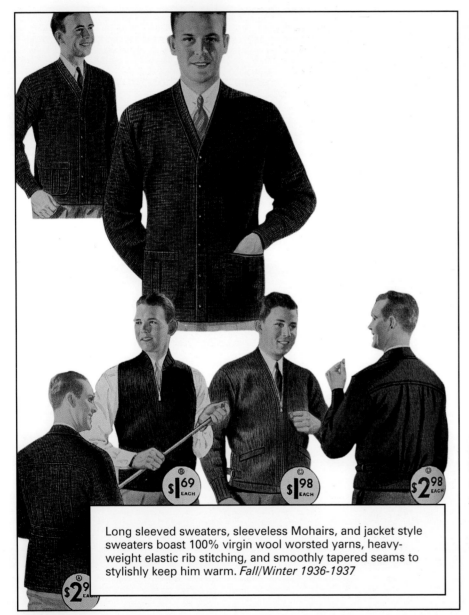

Long sleeved sweaters, sleeveless Mohairs, and jacket style sweaters boast 100% virgin wool worsted yarns, heavy-weight elastic rib stitching, and smoothly tapered seams to stylishly keep him warm. *Fall/Winter 1936-1937*

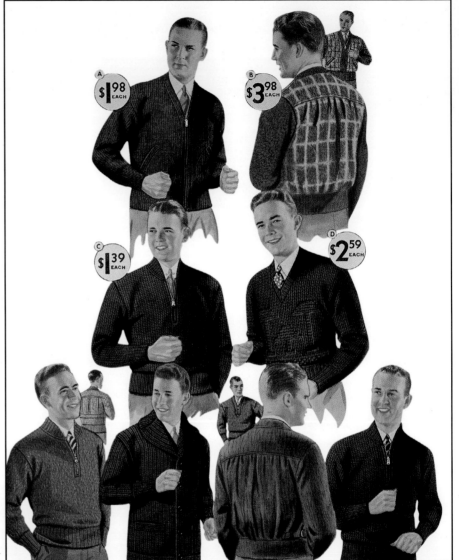

Sporty pullovers, v-necks, button ups, and zippered sweaters are the height of fashion. *Fall/Winter 1936-1937*

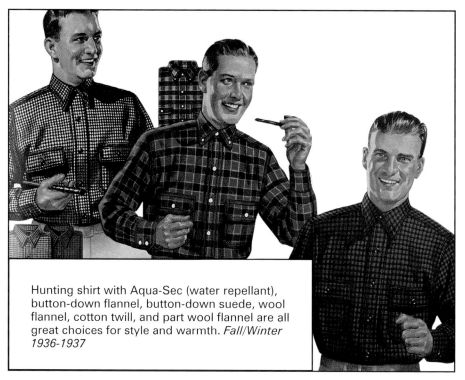

Hunting shirt with Aqua-Sec (water repellant), button-down flannel, button-down suede, wool flannel, cotton twill, and part wool flannel are all great choices for style and warmth. *Fall/Winter 1936-1937*

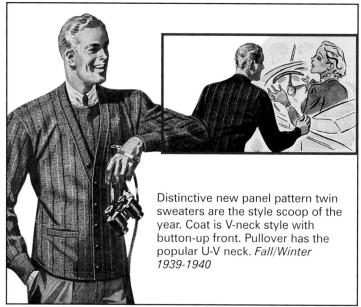

Distinctive new panel pattern twin sweaters are the style scoop of the year. Coat is V-neck style with button-up front. Pullover has the popular U-V neck. *Fall/Winter 1939-1940*

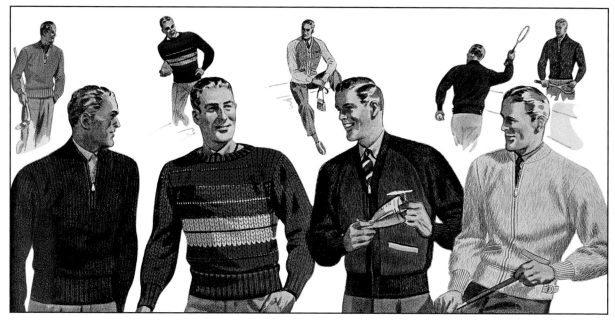

Sweaters for men in fabrics such as wool, wool mohair, and wool/cotton combinations. Styled in Twin Sweaters, pull-over, cardigan, rib knit, solids, and contrasting stripes. *Fall/Winter 1939-1940*

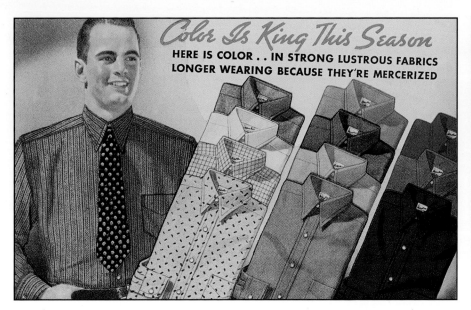

Cotton broadcloth shirts with fused collars that won't wilt or wrinkle. *Fall/Winter 1937-1938*

Army style heavy flannel shirts have a lined chest and double thickness at the elbow. 1/4 wool flannel shirts in zip style or button-up style. *Fall/Winter 1937-1938*

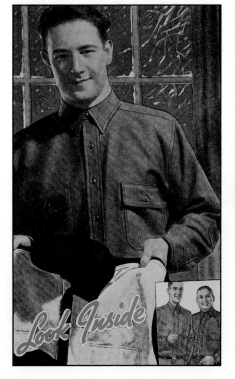

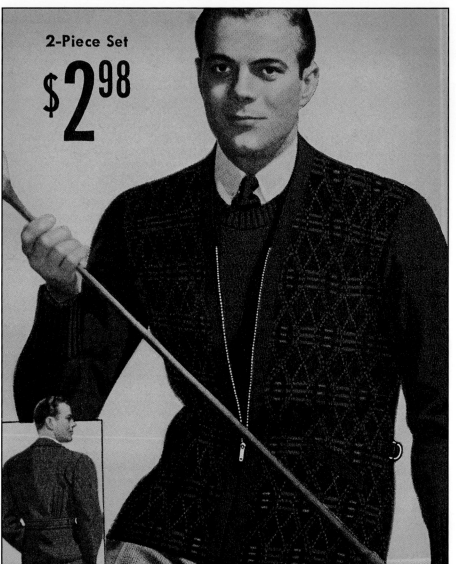

2-piece Twin sweaters are made with Mohair wool, balance cotton and rayon yarns. Sleeveless pullover has a U-neck and is finished in solid color to match back and sleeve of coat. Coat is styled with the swing of a Cossack jacket, with slash pockets and adjustable tabs at the waist. Front is patterned in subdued colors. Very fashionable this year! *Fall/Winter 1937-1938*

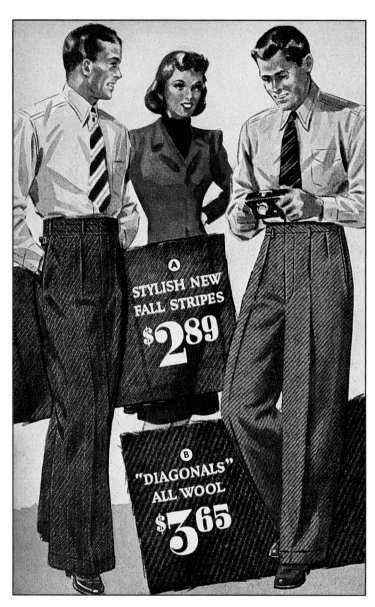

Dressy Collegiate styling in popular green or brown has a handsome striped diagonal weave worsted smooth finish. Full pleats, adjustable side straps, and swaggering 22" cuffs. *Fall/Winter 1939-1940*

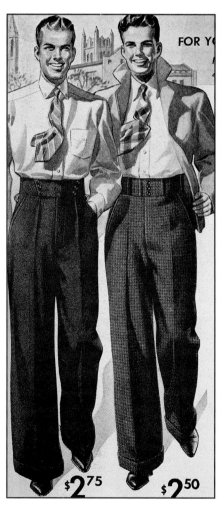

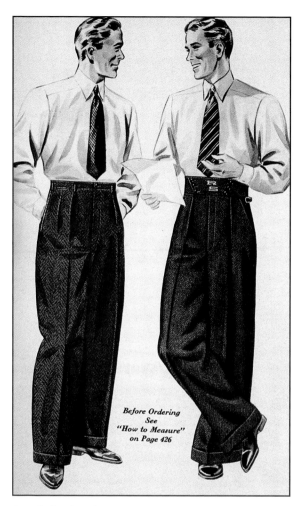

A style leader, these extremely popular wide wale Herringbone All Virgin Wool Worsted have double pleats, fine trimmings, and 20" cuffs. Cheviot in favorite Herringbone weave have fancy 6-button waistband, pleats, 22" cuffs with "Everstay" crease. *Fall/Winter 1939-1940*

Youths and young men will love these high waisted, wide cuffed trousers. Available in Dark Blue, Oxford, Gray Check, and Brown Check. *Fall/Winter 1936-1937*

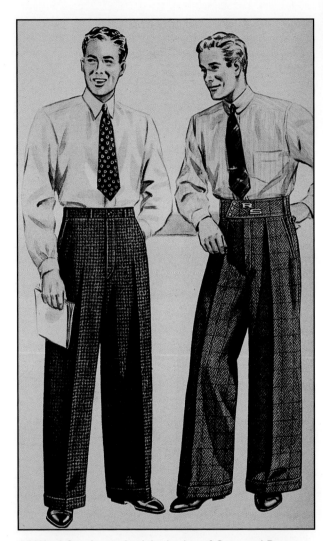

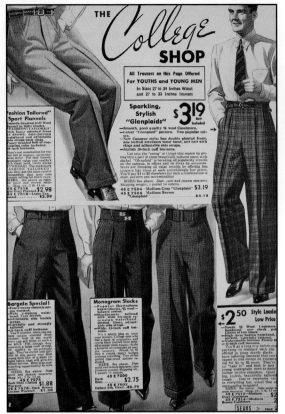

The College Shop's fashion tailored sports flannel trousers have a fancy stitch sewn on front with fancy braided belt. "Glenplaids" are wool Cassimere, double pleated front, and self-belt. Fancy weave smooth cotton worsted tailored trousers has a wide 3-button waistband and 21" cuff bottoms. Monogrammed slacks in Herringbone weave with tailored 3-1/2" extension waistband, pleated front, and 22" cuff bottoms. Wool Cassimere in check patter, high 3-button waistband, 21" cuff bottoms. *Spring/Summer 1937*

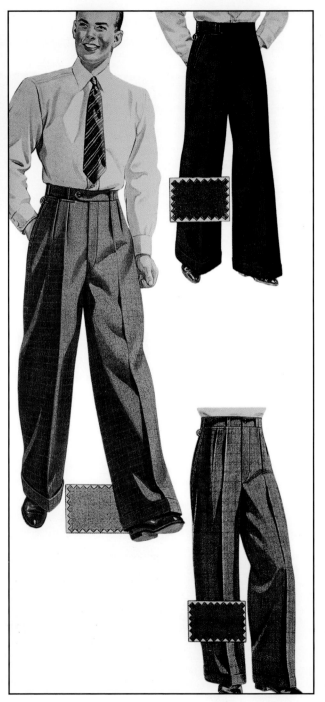

All Wool Cassimere in rich shades of Gray and Brown, 1-button model-side straps, and 20" cuffs. Smooth Cassimere in herringbone with overplaid has 5-button extension waistband, adjustable side straps, and 2 initials included with these dressy slacks. *Fall/Winter 1939-1940*

Assorted men's Fashion Tailored slacks in all the latest styles and colors. *Spring/Summer 1937*

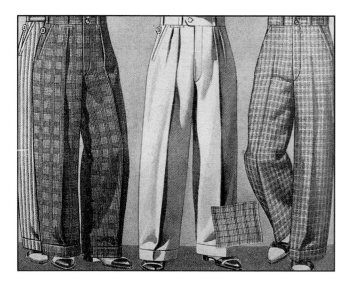

Pleated slacks for a sporty or dressy look in neat summer patterns and colors. *Spring/Summer 1938*

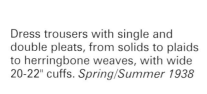

Dress trousers with single and double pleats, from solids to plaids to herringbone weaves, with wide 20-22" cuffs. *Spring/Summer 1938*

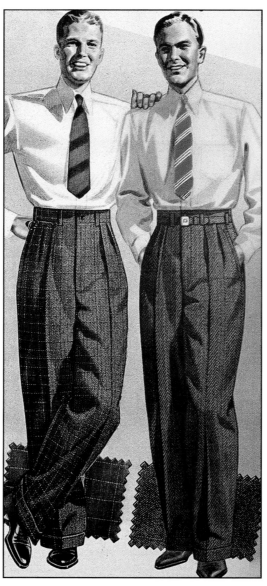

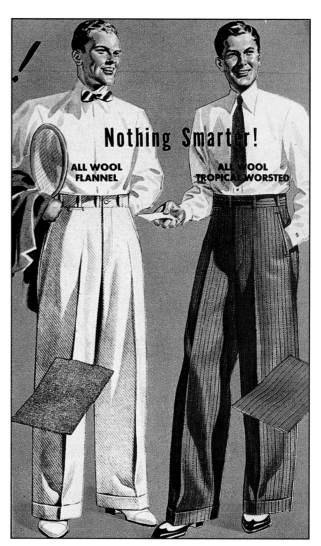

Nothing Smarter!

ALL WOOL FLANNEL

ALL WOOL TROPICAL WORSTED

All Wool flannel trousers are always in and look good alone or with a dark coat. All Wool Tropical Worsted are cool and hold their drapery fit. *Spring/Summer 1938*

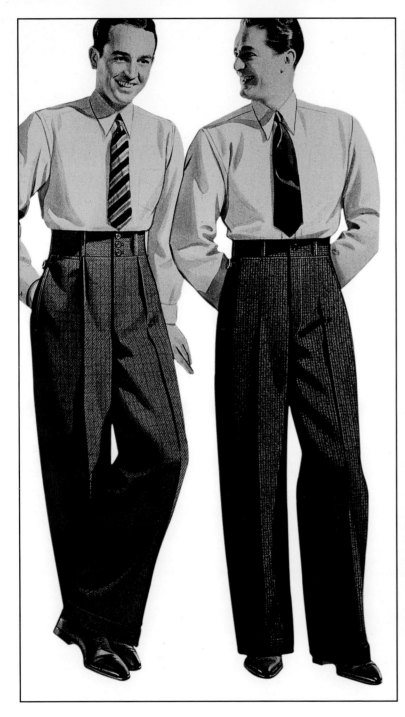

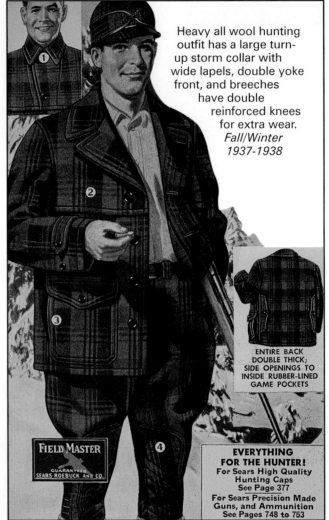

Heavy all wool hunting outfit has a large turn-up storm collar with wide lapels, double yoke front, and breeches have double reinforced knees for extra wear. *Fall/Winter 1937-1938*

ENTIRE BACK DOUBLE THICK; SIDE OPENINGS TO INSIDE RUBBER-LINED GAME POCKETS

FIELD MASTER
GUARANTEED
SEARS ROEBUCK AND CO.

EVERYTHING FOR THE HUNTER!
For Sears High Quality Hunting Caps See Page 377
For Sears Precision Made Guns, and Ammunition See Pages 748 to 753

Popular check pattern with overplaid trousers have snappy pleated front, a wide 3" waistband, side straps and rings. All wool cassimere check pattern trousers with conventional styling, a 1-button waistband, adjustable side straps, and regular 20" cuff bottoms. *Fall/Winter 1937-1938*

Sleepwear/Underwear

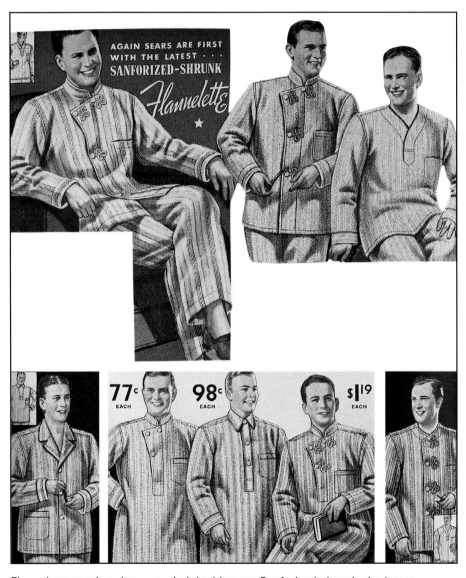

Flannelette men's pajamas and nightshirts are Sanforized-shrunk, the latest technique to ensure no shrinking. *Fall/Winter 1936-1937*

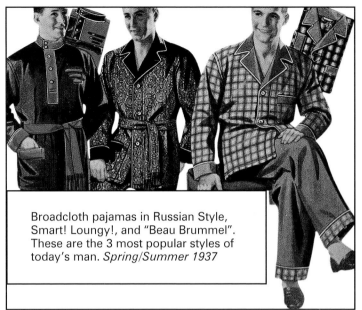

Broadcloth pajamas in Russian Style, Smart! Loungy!, and "Beau Brummel". These are the 3 most popular styles of today's man. *Spring/Summer 1937*

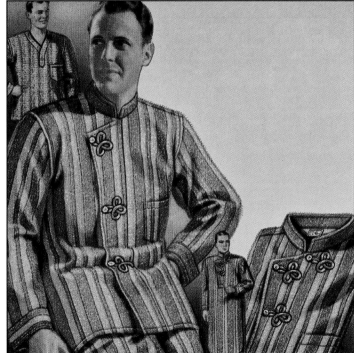

Flannelette pajamas and nightshirt with military collar and frog-trimmed buttonholes. *Fall/Winter 1937-1938*

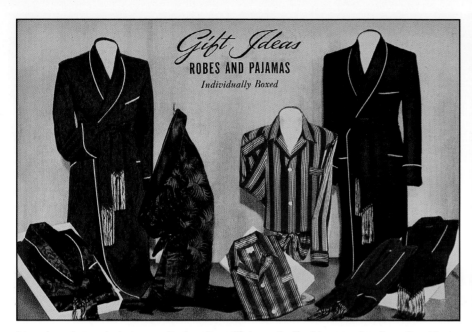

Luxurious brocaded rayon robe in a beautiful scroll effect jacquard pattern lined in silk. Soft brocaded rayon robe in jacquard pattern looks and feels like real silk. Crown tested rayon pajamas has the costly softness of silk. De Luxe Wool Flannel wrap around robe trimmed with contrasting color piped edges. *Fall/Winter 1939-1940*

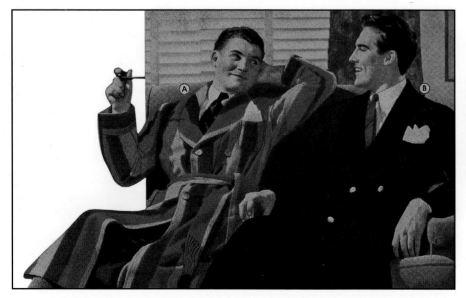

Men's robes in many styles and patterns including Ombre, plaids, stripes, and two-tones. *Fall/Winter 1938/1939*

Genuine "St. Moritz" all wool flannel robes with double stitched seams and contrasting pearl buttons in wide stripes or solid colors. *Fall/Winter 1937-1938*

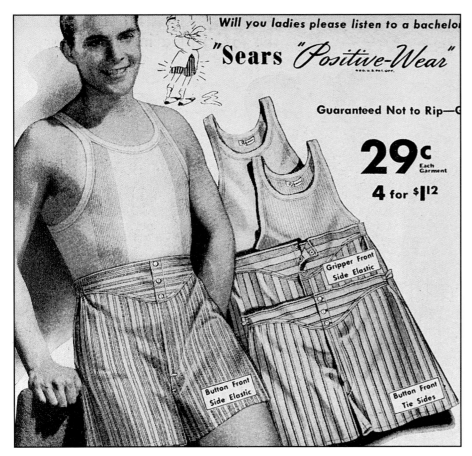

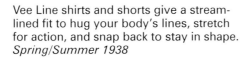

Positive-Wear shorts are guaranteed not to shrink or tear and Kilburn combed cotton shirts are soft and comfortable. *Fall/Winter 1939-1940*

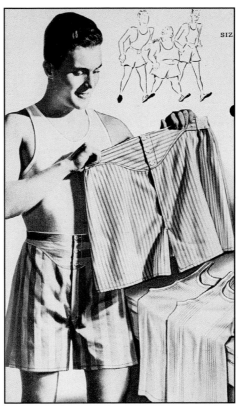

"Positive Wear" shorts are guaranteed to be the strongest you can buy because the seams are triple stitched, bartacked at stress points, and the crotch is doubled. Fancy patterns or White. *Spring/Summer 1939*

Vee Line shirts and shorts give a streamlined fit to hug your body's lines, stretch for action, and snap back to stay in shape. *Spring/Summer 1938*

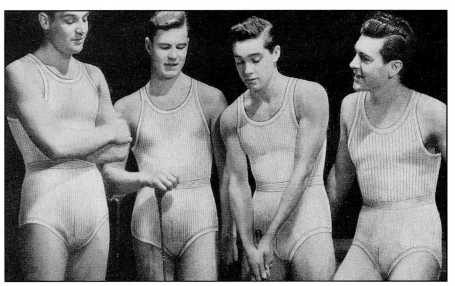

Men's underwear in styles for short, medium, and tall men. *Spring/Summer 1938*

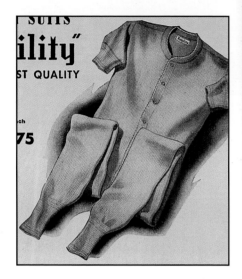

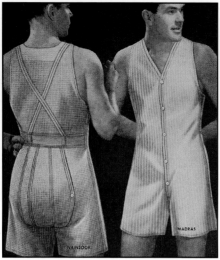

Union Suits underwear. If you are tall and slim, short and stout, or of average build, there are styles and fits just for you. *Fall/Winter 1939-1940*

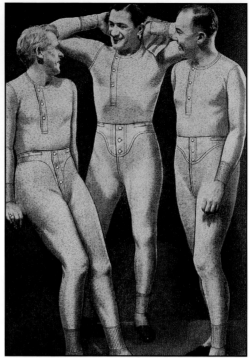

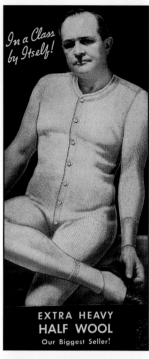

EXTRA HEAVY
HALF WOOL
Our Biggest Seller!

Vee Lines offer no bulk, no weight, no buttons on their underwear in sleeveless shirt/shorts, 3/4-length longs and short sleeve shirt, and ankle length longs with short sleeve shirt. *Fall/Winter 1939-1940*

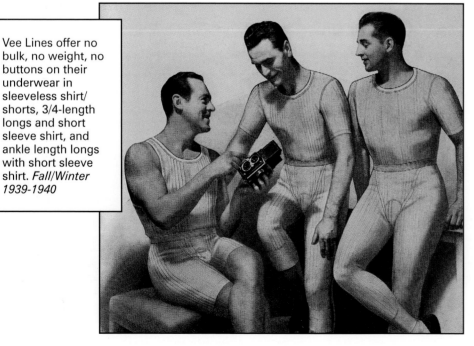

Pilgrim wool underwear are warm and comfortable for cold winter days. Shirts and drawers are tailored with the softest wool yarns, are roomy, and will not bind. Ankle length drawers have adjustable tie-back and ribbed anklets, shirts have ribbed bottoms and cuffs. *Fall/Winter 1938/1939*

Top right:
Extra heavy half wool/cotton suit is elastic spring needle knit to keep its fit, has inset shoulders that won't sag, collarette neck fits comfortable, and cuffs and anklets are snugly ribbed. *Fall/Winter 1937-1938*

Long sleeve shirts and ankle length drawers are heavy weight and warm. *Fall/Winter 1937-1938*

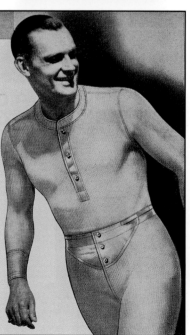

Outerwear

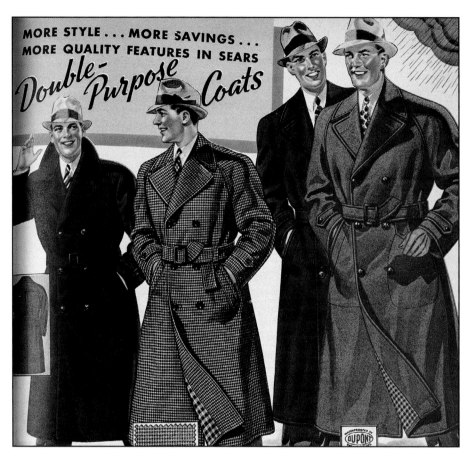

"Rain-O-Shine" and "Buckskein" men's coats are made of splendid quality. All are 48" long and the "Buckskein" is guaranteed windproof and waterproof. *Fall/Winter 1936-1937*

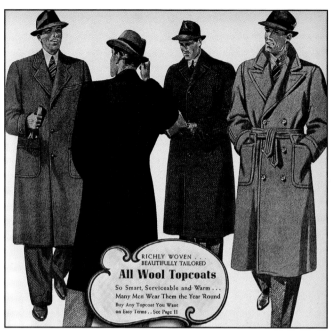

All Wool Topcoats in Herringbone Cheviot, the popular "Guards" model in herringbone pattern with overplaid, new diagonal tweeds in Green or Brown, and the debonair Camel Tan "Polo". *Fall/Winter 1939-1940*

Exclusively at Sears, the nationally famous Buckskein coats for men are waterproof, windproof, wear-tested, and warm. *Fall/Winter 1939-1940*

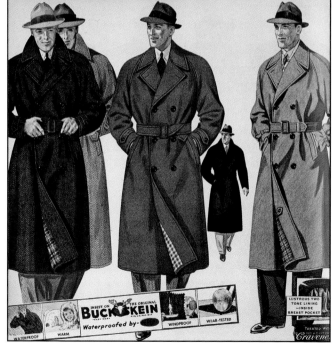

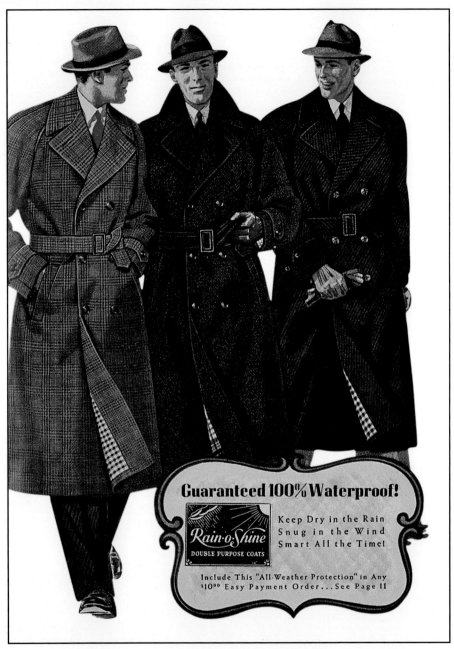

Rain-o-Shine coats for men are waterproof and found in Suede-texture, herringbone, diagonals, or reversible styles. *Fall/Winter 1939-1940*

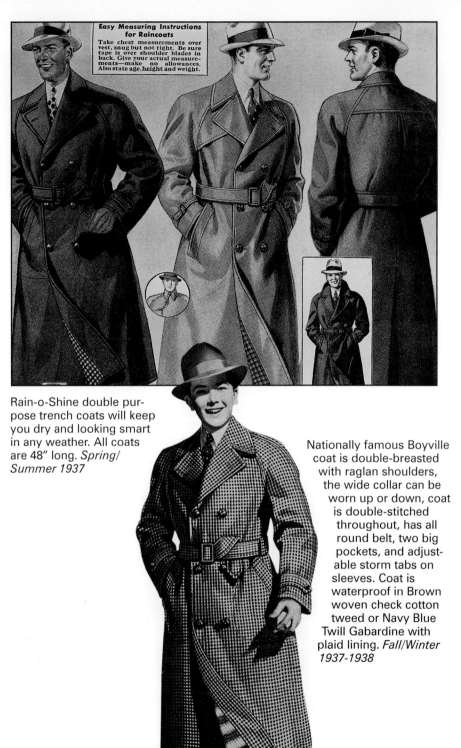

Easy Measuring Instructions for Raincoats
Take chest measurements over vest, snug but not tight. Be sure tape is over shoulder blades in back. Give your actual measurements—make no allowances. Also state age, height and weight.

Rain-o-Shine double purpose trench coats will keep you dry and looking smart in any weather. All coats are 48" long. *Spring/ Summer 1937*

Nationally famous Boyville coat is double-breasted with raglan shoulders, the wide collar can be worn up or down, coat is double-stitched throughout, has all round belt, two big pockets, and adjustable storm tabs on sleeves. Coat is waterproof in Brown woven check cotton tweed or Navy Blue Twill Gabardine with plaid lining. *Fall/Winter 1937-1938*

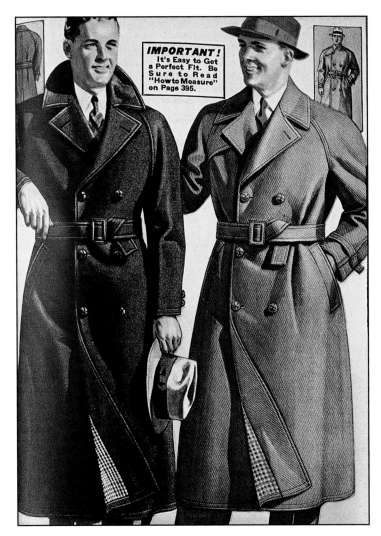

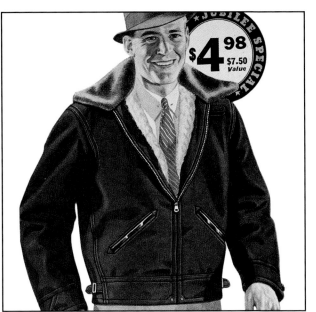

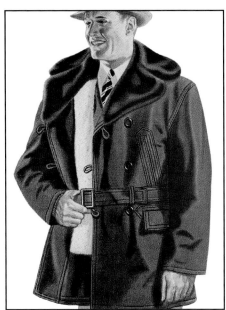

Men's coats feature sheepskin lining with either Wide Wale Corduroy or Moleskin. *Fall/Winter 1936-1937*

Rain-O-Shine double-breasted polo coat is suede-like and smooth as velvet, has leather buttons and buckles, wide collar, and is always in good taste. Double-breasted Trench coat in tan cotton twill Gabardine vulcanized with pure gum rubber to a fast color plaid cotton lining, has raglan sleeves and big roomy pockets. *Fall/Winter 1937-1938*

Men's coats of cotton suede, and a fleecy mohair finished fabric with several layers of pure gum rubber. *Fall/Winter 1936-1937*

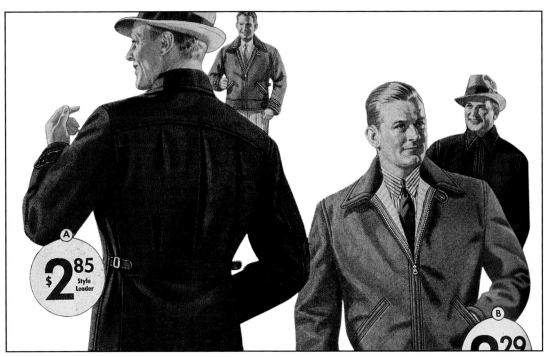

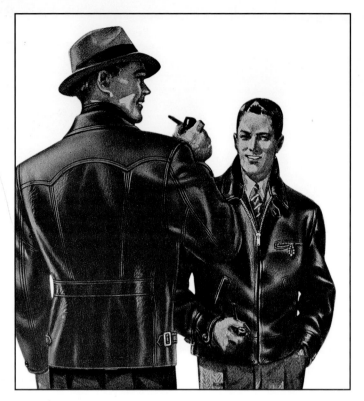

Horsehide jackets are windproof, crackproof, and scuffproof, in all the latest styles. Jackets are lined with fancy plaid wool, durable corduroy, or cotton flannel. *Fall/Winter 1939-1940*

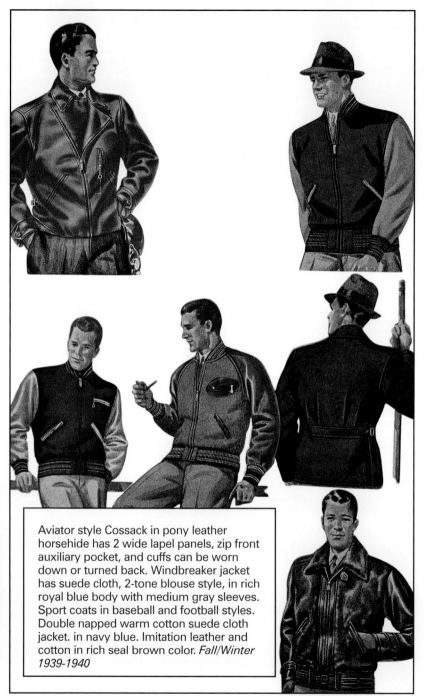

Sporty leather jackets uses select skins, has rayon lining, are good looking and comfortable to wear. *Fall/Winter 1939-1940*

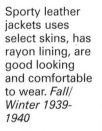

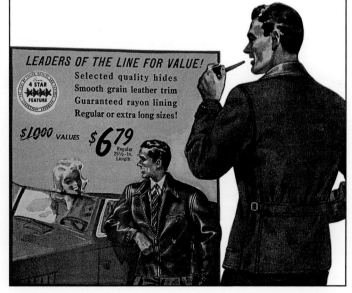

LEADERS OF THE LINE FOR VALUE!
Selected quality hides
Smooth grain leather trim
Guaranteed rayon lining
Regular or extra long sizes!

4 STAR FEATURE

$10.00 VALUES $6.79
Regular
25½-In.
Length

Aviator style Cossack in pony leather horsehide has 2 wide lapel panels, zip front auxiliary pocket, and cuffs can be worn down or turned back. Windbreaker jacket has suede cloth, 2-tone blouse style, in rich royal blue body with medium gray sleeves. Sport coats in baseball and football styles. Double napped warm cotton suede cloth jacket. in navy blue. Imitation leather and cotton in rich seal brown color. *Fall/Winter 1939-1940*

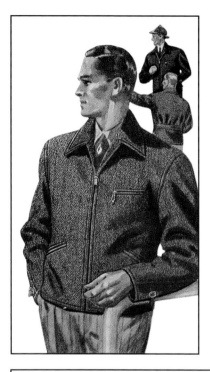

Buckskein jackets have zip fronts, are rainproof, windproof, and warm. *Fall/Winter 1939-1940*

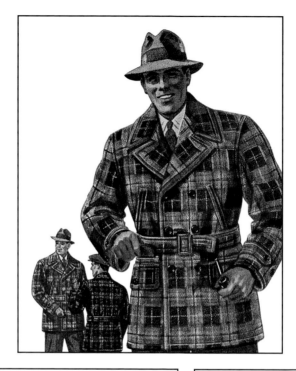

Sears Four Star Feature coat in plaid. Border Stripe in Blue or Green, Lustrous Silvertone in Maroon or Blue, and Railroader in Oxford Gray or Navy Blue. *Fall/Winter 1939-1940*

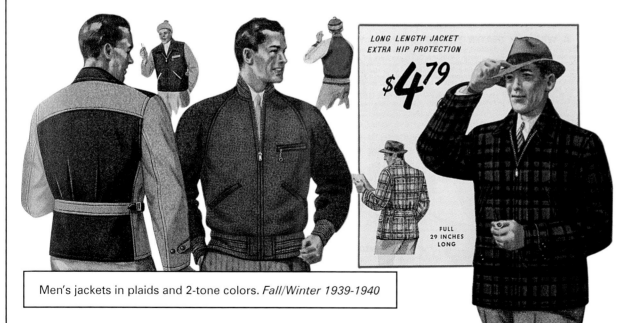

LONG LENGTH JACKET
EXTRA HIP PROTECTION

$4.79

FULL 29 INCHES LONG

Men's jackets in plaids and 2-tone colors. *Fall/Winter 1939-1940*

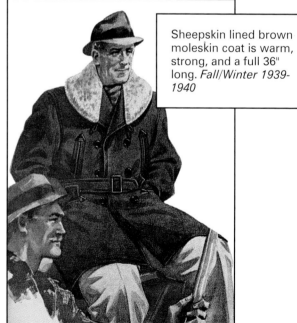

Sheepskin lined brown moleskin coat is warm, strong, and a full 36" long. *Fall/Winter 1939-1940*

Shoes

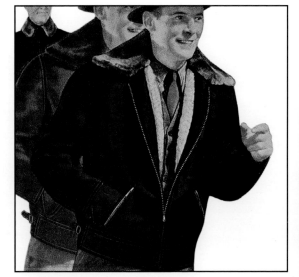

Hercules sheep lined horsehide and corduroy coats with fur-lined collars. *Fall/Winter 1939-1940*

Sheepskin lined jackets for action, warmth, and wear. *Fall/Winter 1937-1938*

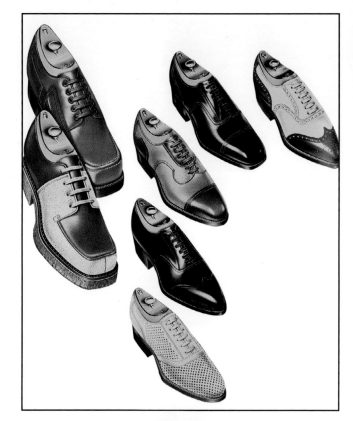

Sporty "Box Cars", Smart Summer Brogues, Stylish French Toes, Sporty new Two-Tones, Short Wing Tips, and Ventilated Leather Uppers are high style. *Spring/Summer 1939*

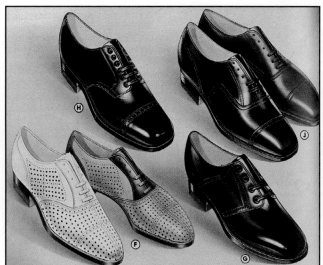

Bob Burnham fine calfskin thrift shoes in smart and sporty styles. *Spring/Summer 1938*

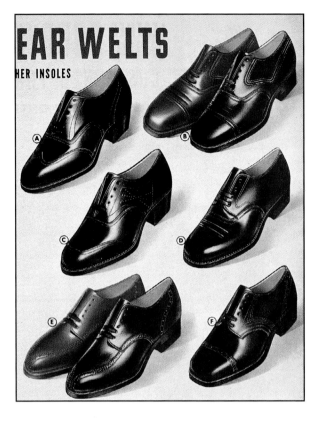

EAR WELTS

HER INSOLES

Goodyear welts have smooth, one-piece solid leather insoles, fully lined for comfort, and are easy on your feet. *Fall/Winter 1938/1939*

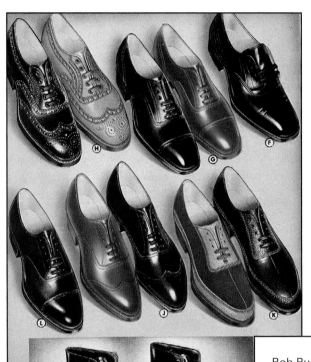

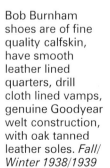

Bob Burnham shoes are of fine quality calfskin, have smooth leather lined quarters, drill cloth lined vamps, genuine Goodyear welt construction, with oak tanned leather soles. *Fall/Winter 1938/1939*

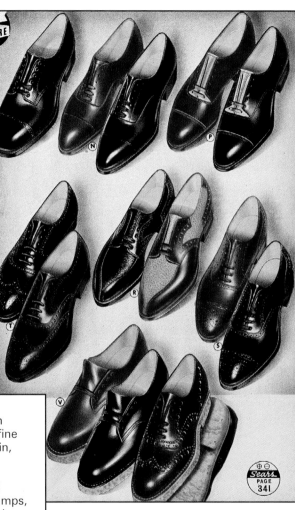

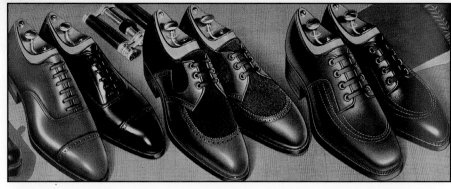

Gold Bonds are equal to any other with the finest quality select leather uppers, oak-tanned bend leather outsoles, grain leather insoles, calfskin lined quarters, Goodyear Welt construction, and white drill cloth lined vamps. *Fall/Winter 1937-1938*

Sears finest shoes are made on modern, fine-fitting lasts by skilled craftsmen with the finest quality oak-tanned bend leather outsoles, genuine Goodyear Welts, sturdy sole leather counters, buffed leather insoles, and smooth calfskin lined quarters. *Fall/Winter 1937-1938*

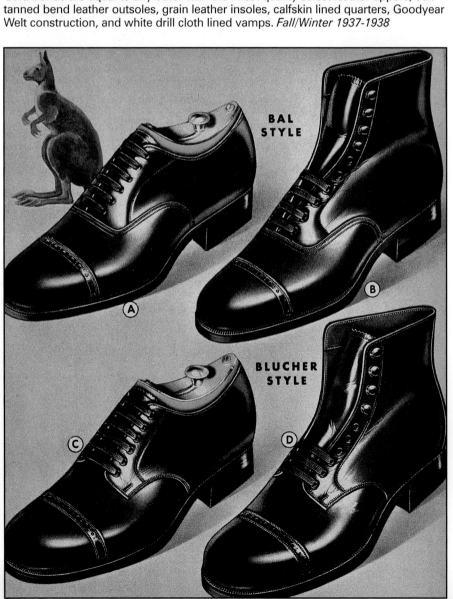

BAL STYLE

BLUCHER STYLE

Sears Kangaroo leather is tougher and stronger than any other leather known, yet is amazingly pliable and soft as an "old-slipper". It's tight, even grain takes a high, lustrous polish so necessary for that smart, well-groomed appearance. *Fall/Winter 1937-1938*

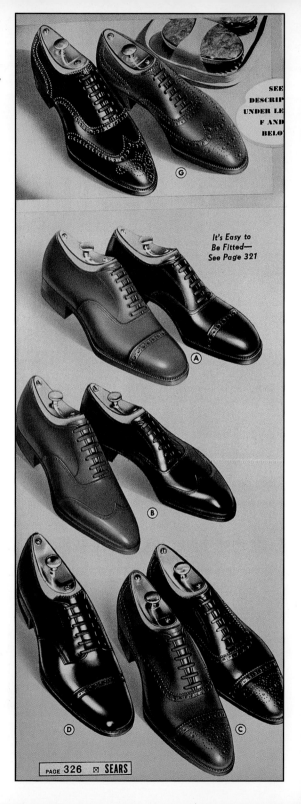

SEE DESCRIP UNDER LE F AND BELO

It's Easy to Be Fitted— See Page 321

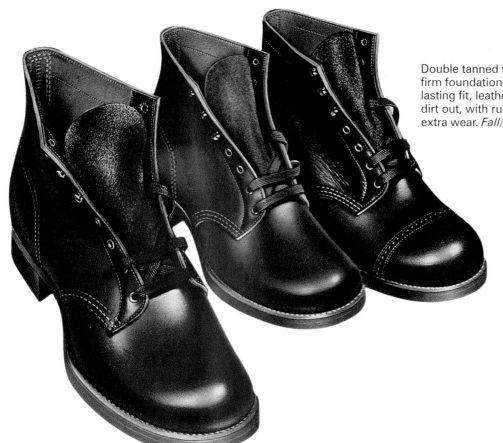

Double tanned farm shoes have firm foundations for comfort and lasting fit, leather tongs keeps dirt out, with rubber heels for extra wear. *Fall/Winter 1939-1940*

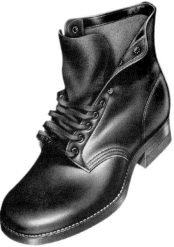

Sears Good Lucks are made of cordovan-type horsehide, the toughest, most pliable leather tanned. Chrome-tanned elk-grained cowhide leather uppers are comfortable with orthopedic type rubber heel and steel shank to provide extra arch support. "Shockless" boots have inside arch lift for support, sponge rubber shock-absorber insole, and built-in steel shank to hold up arches. *Fall/Winter 1937-1938*

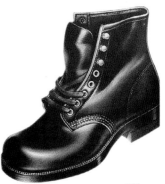

Men's boots of quality with leather covered cushion insoles, firm leather insole bases, Steinbrecher steel arch supports, genuine Goodyear welts, oak-tanned bend leather soles, and Goodyear wing foot rubber heels. *Spring/Summer 1939*

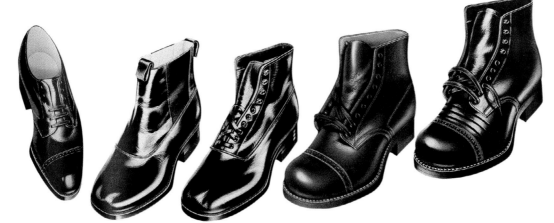

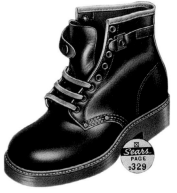

Sears
PAGE
329

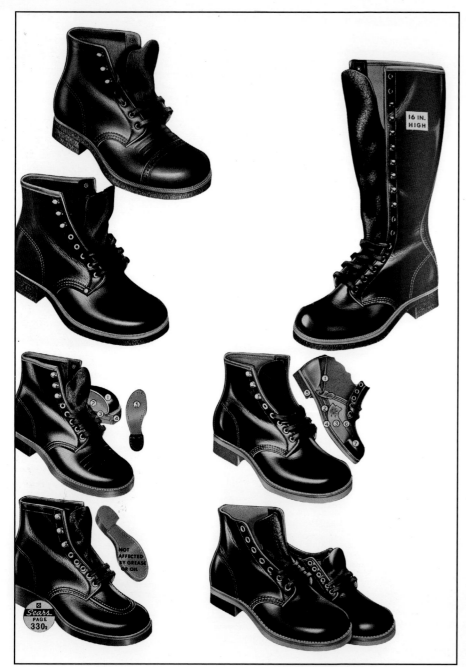

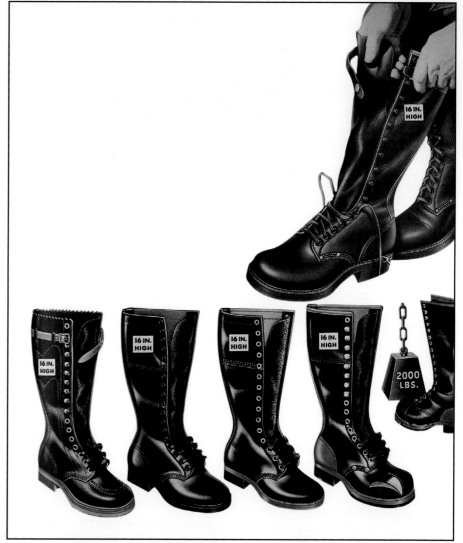

Husky Hi-Cuts in Grain Leather with patented adjustable snap and strap, Moccasin Style toe with 13-nail rubber heel, Double tanned black leather uppers, Solid leather uppers, and heavy steel toe in double tanned black leather. *Fall/Winter 1937-1938*

Brown cap toe style boots, black with plain toe, husky hi-cuts, black elk-grain leather uppers, double tanned boots, "Rock Oak" , and non-marking "Compo" soled boots. *Fall/Winter 1937-1938*

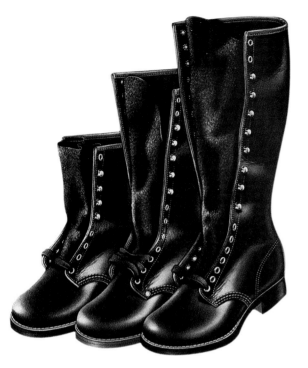

Oil tanned boots resist moisture better than any other leather you can buy. These boots are great for farming, logging, or any tough job that demands sturdiness. *Fall/Winter 1938/1939*

Oil tanned dark brown leather uppers from 6" to 16" high. Solid leather work shoes are acid-resistant by the double-tanning process, and have 13-nail rubber heel. Double-tanned leather upper with genuine Goodyear Welt construction. *Fall/Winter 1937-1938*

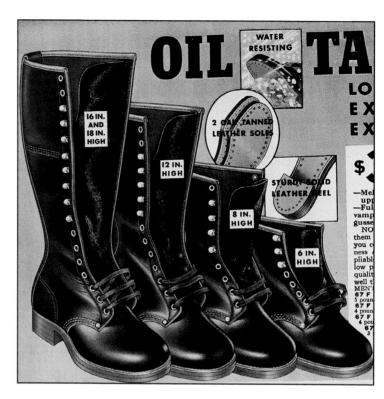

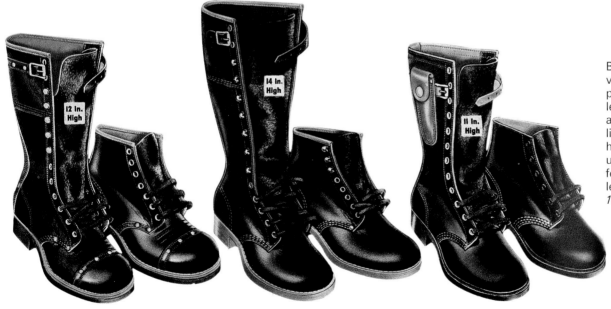

Black split leather uppers with strongly riveted toe cap, vamp, and back strap, heavy "Compo" outsole and one-piece oak-leather mid-sole nailed and sewed. Oil-tanned leather uppers with oak tanned bend leather outsoles and oak-tanned leather midsoles, nailed and sewed, drill lined vamps triple stitched with harness thread, and heavy nickel hooks and eyelets. Black split leather uppers of heavy "Compo" outsole brass plated nailed for greater wear, rubber storm welt, one-piece grain leather insole, and leather gusset tongue. *Fall/Winter 1937-1938*

133

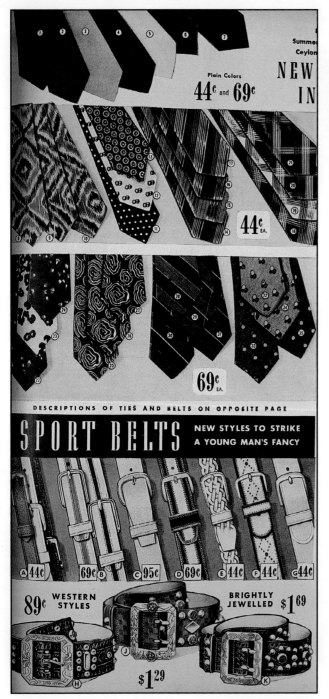

Accessories

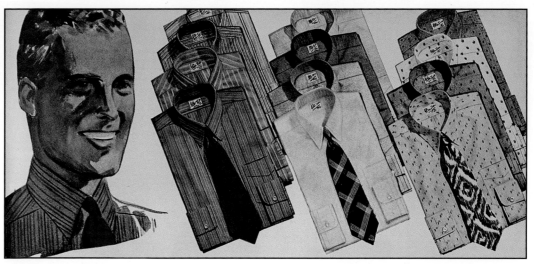

Fashion Tower shirts and ties are tailored in high-count cotton fabrics with roomy dimensions. They are Sanforized, Vat-dyed, with Non-Wilt fused collars. *Spring/Summer 1939*

A man never has too many belts! *Fall/Winter 1938/1939*

Stylish ties and belts for the modern man. *Spring/Summer 1939*

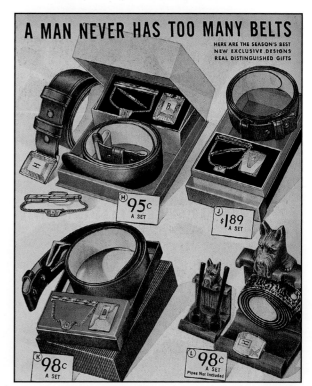

Teen Boys

Suits

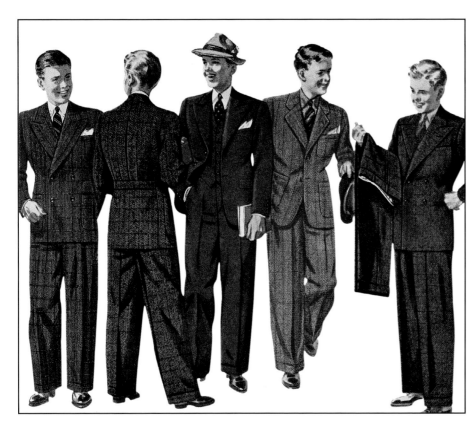

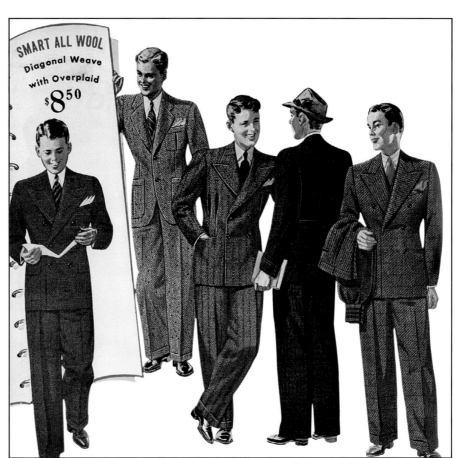

All Wool boy's suits in the famous "Fraternity Prep" style. Shown with single and double-breasted jackets. *Fall/Winter 1939-1940*

Man styled suits for older boys. *Fall/Winter 1939-1940*

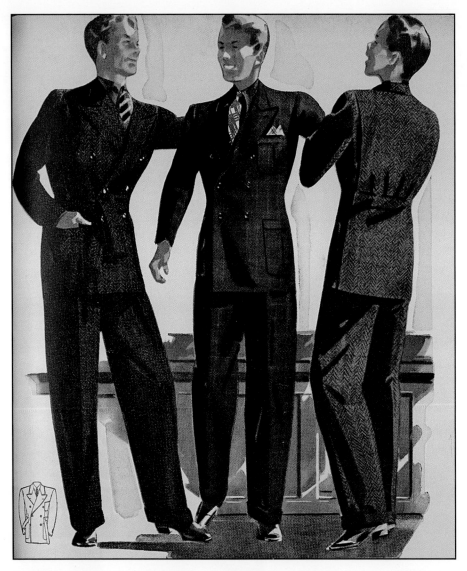

Double-breasted suits in herringbone weave or overplaids The suits are All Wool and come in styles that set the pace! *Spring/Summer 1939*

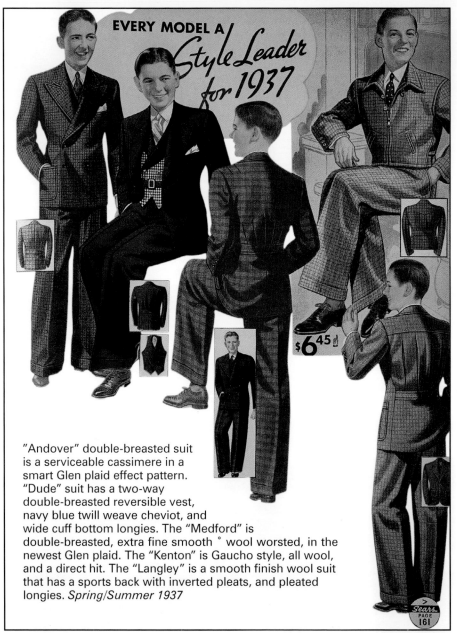

6^{45}

"Andover" double-breasted suit is a serviceable cassimere in a smart Glen plaid effect pattern. "Dude" suit has a two-way double-breasted reversible vest, navy blue twill weave cheviot, and wide cuff bottom longies. The "Medford" is double-breasted, extra fine smooth ° wool worsted, in the newest Glen plaid. The "Kenton" is Gaucho style, all wool, and a direct hit. The "Langley" is a smooth finish wool suit that has a sports back with inverted pleats, and pleated longies. *Spring/Summer 1937*

Sears PAGE 161

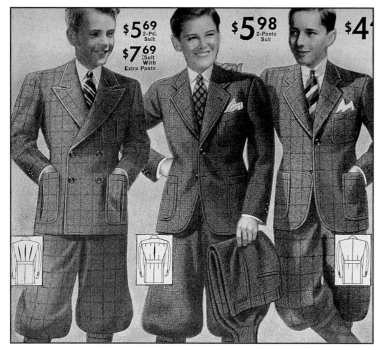

Knicker suits for young men
in popular plaids and solids
are right for any occasion.
Spring/Summer 1938

Fraternity Prep all wool suits in smooth weave with overplaid, herringbone with subdued overplaid, and subdued stripes. Very smart. *Fall/Winter 1938/1939*

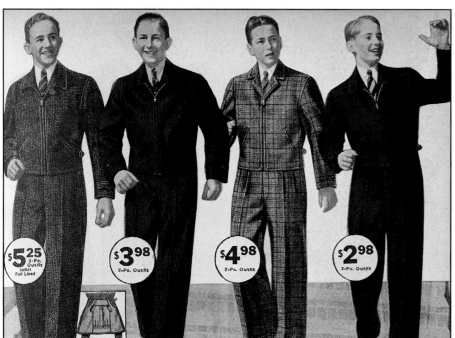

Two-piece outfits in corduroy and part-wool fabrics. *Fall/Winter 1937-1938*

Casual

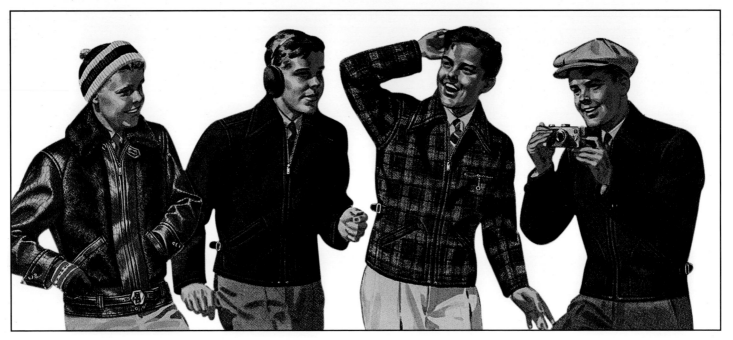

Boy's sports jackets in plaids, solids, leather, and wool and leather combinations. *Fall/Winter 1939-1940*

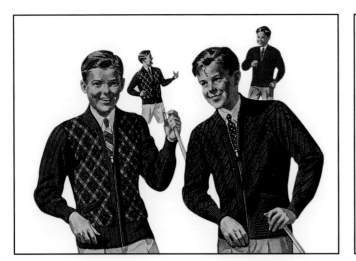
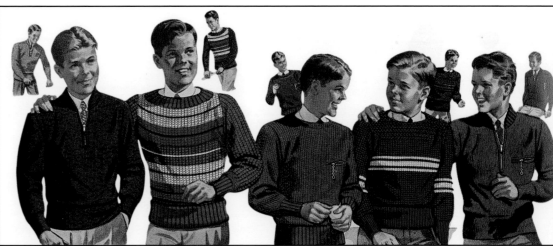

All Wool Worsted sporty zip front sweaters, the new barrel neck cardigan stitched sweater, Wool crew neck, sturdy cardigan stitched, and napped wool with zip opening. *Fall/Winter 1939-1940*

Raglan style twin sweater in soft napped All Wool zip front coat with zip chest pocket. Royal blue with gray or maroon with gray. *Fall/Winter 1939-1940*

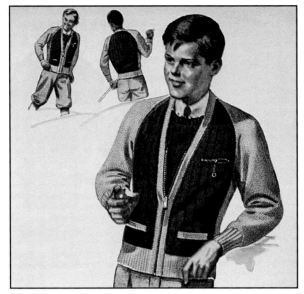

Rugged corduroy campus favorites for boys are warm for outdoor activities. *Fall/Winter 1939-1940*

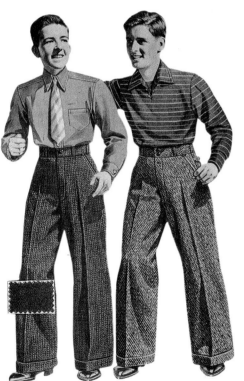

Inexpensive and dressy slacks in brown check cassimere or navy blue twill cheviot have one-button waistband, four strong pockets, and wide cuff bottoms. Blouse is dark blue cotton broadcloth. Sturdy Tweed slacks in brown or gray have four twill pockets and wide cuff bottoms. Dark Blue striped cotton jersey knit Polo blouse. *Fall/Winter 1937-1938*

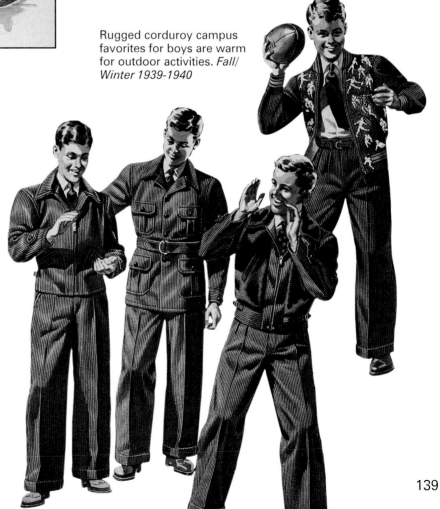

139

Outerwear

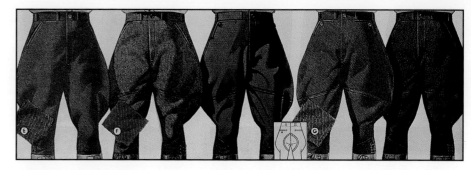

Breeches for active boys are strong and durable, warm, and full cut for comfort. *Fall/Winter 1939-1940*

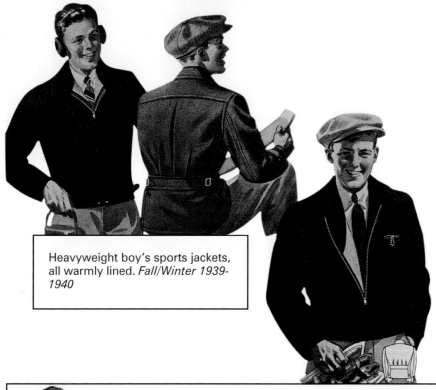

Heavyweight boy's sports jackets, all warmly lined. *Fall/Winter 1939-1940*

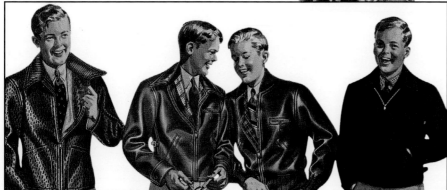

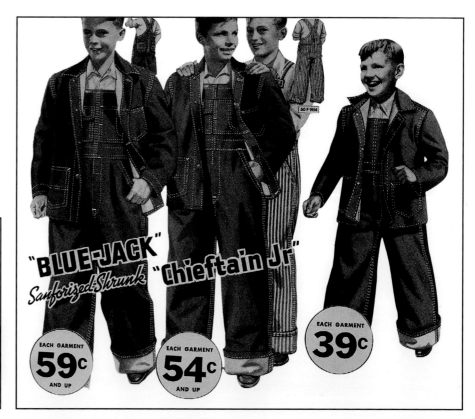

"Blue-Jack" overalls are Sanforized-shrunk, full cut, extra heavy weight denim with no-curl suspenders. "Chieftain Jr" overalls in blue denim or express stripe are cut large and roomy, have wide suspenders and rustproof buckles. Both have matching coats. *Fall/Winter 1937-1938*

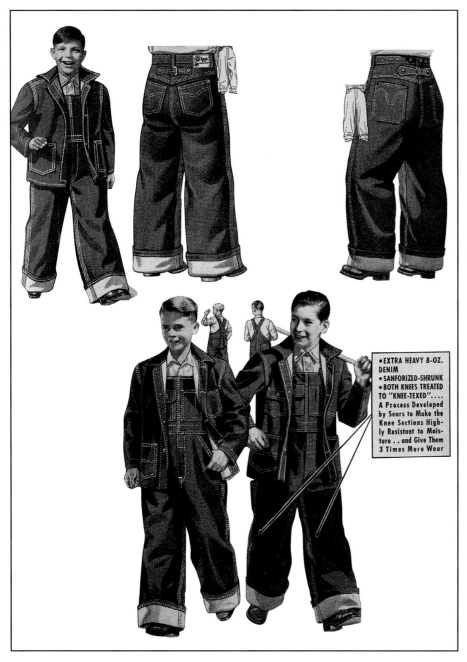

Medium, heavy, and extra heavy denim jackets, pants, and bibs for boy's gives amazing wear. *Fall/Winter 1938/1939*

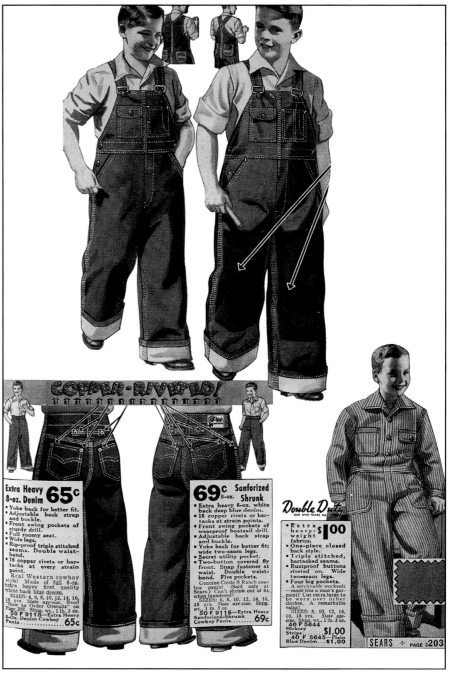

Boys heavy denim overalls, pants, and one-piece suits are strong and long wearing. *Fall/Winter 1937-1938*

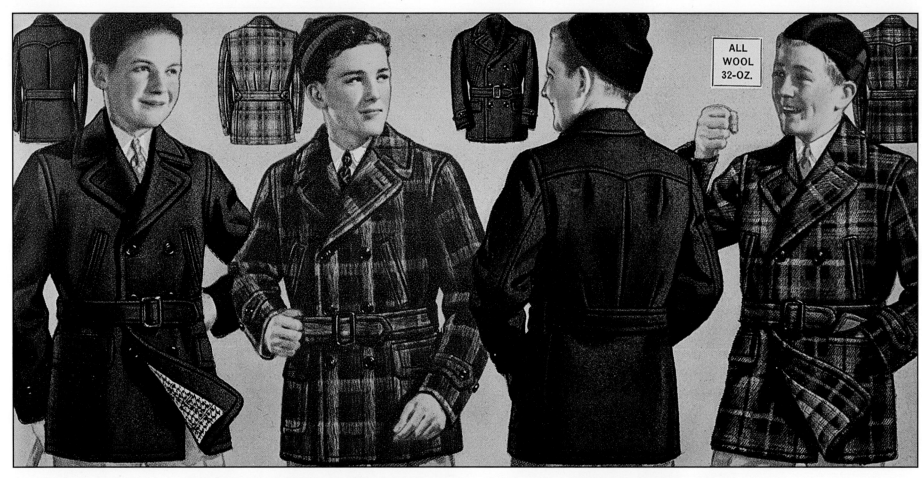

Extra heavy all wool Melton cloth is double breasted, cut full and roomy, fully lined with plaid cotton flannel, and all around belt. Plaid Mackinaw is extra heavy wool, double breasted, in bright new plaids. Wool Melton Mackinaw is extra heavy, has sports back, and is thick and warm. Wool Mackinaw in plaid is water repellent, has flannel lining, sports back, and all around belt. *Fall/Winter 1938/1939*

Accessories

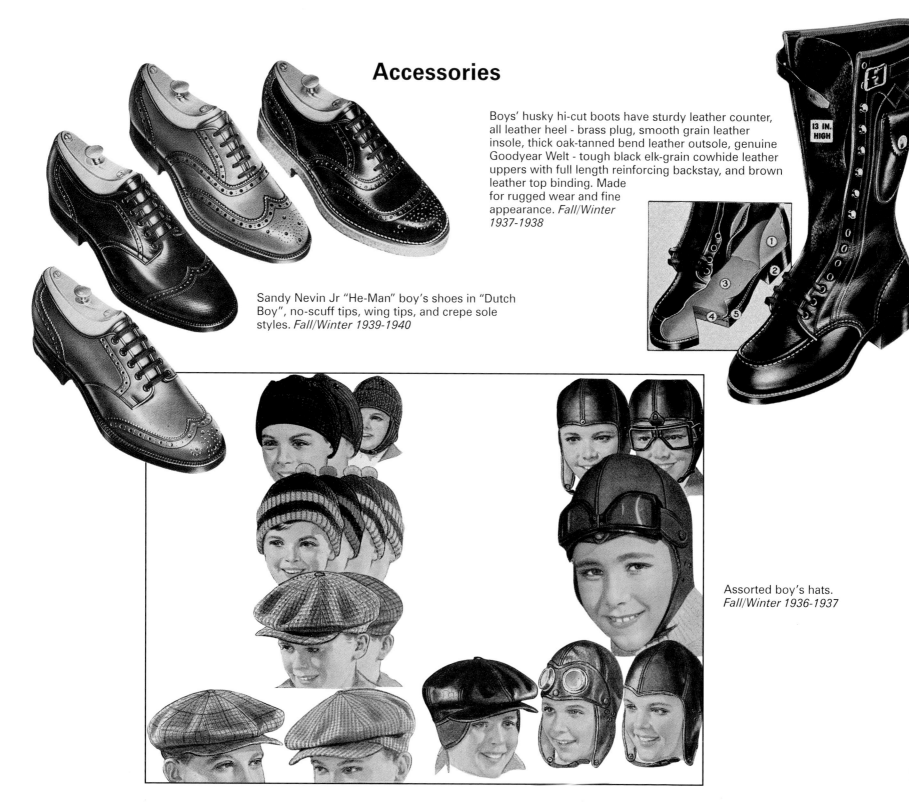

Boys' husky hi-cut boots have sturdy leather counter, all leather heel - brass plug, smooth grain leather insole, thick oak-tanned bend leather outsole, genuine Goodyear Welt - tough black elk-grain cowhide leather uppers with full length reinforcing backstay, and brown leather top binding. Made for rugged wear and fine appearance. *Fall/Winter 1937-1938*

Sandy Nevin Jr "He-Man" boy's shoes in "Dutch Boy", no-scuff tips, wing tips, and crepe sole styles. *Fall/Winter 1939-1940*

Assorted boy's hats. *Fall/Winter 1936-1937*

143

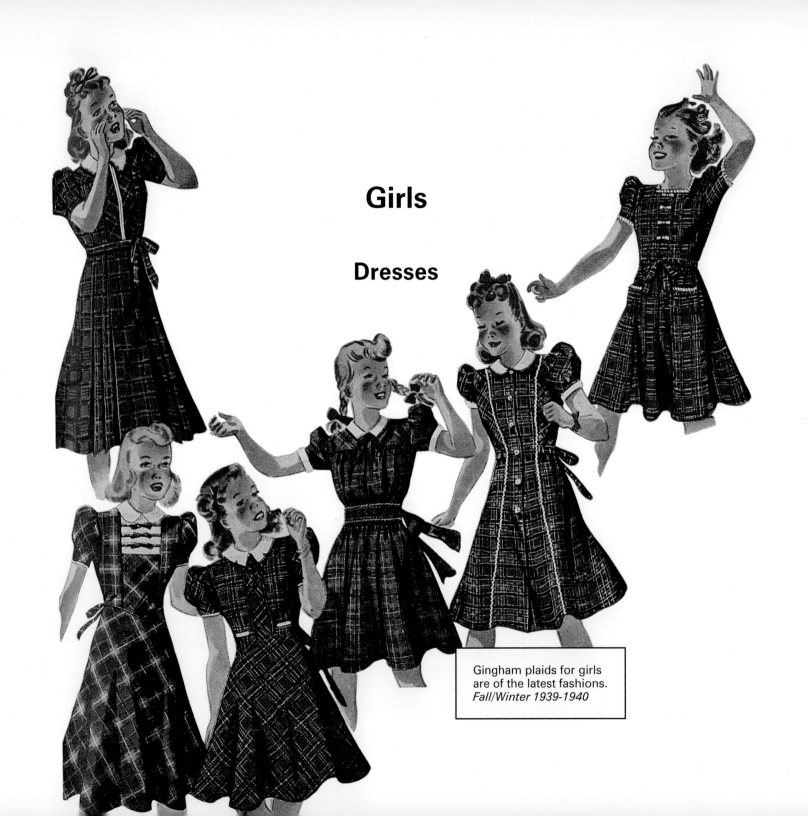

Girls

Dresses

Gingham plaids for girls
are of the latest fashions.
Fall/Winter 1939-1940

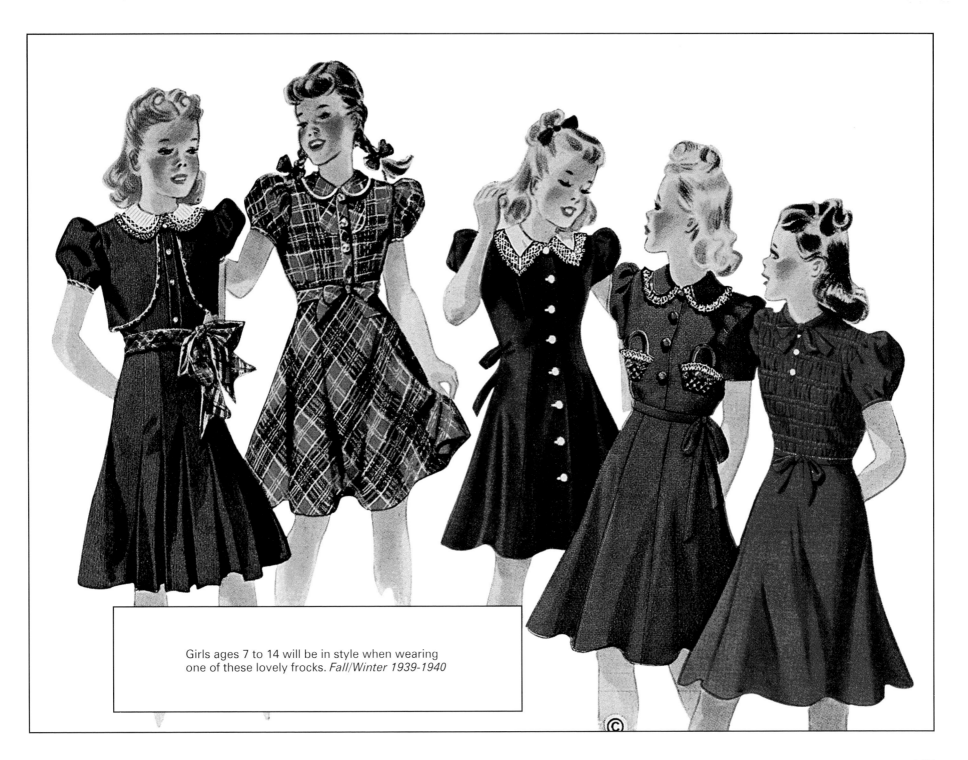

Girls ages 7 to 14 will be in style when wearing one of these lovely frocks. *Fall/Winter 1939-1940*

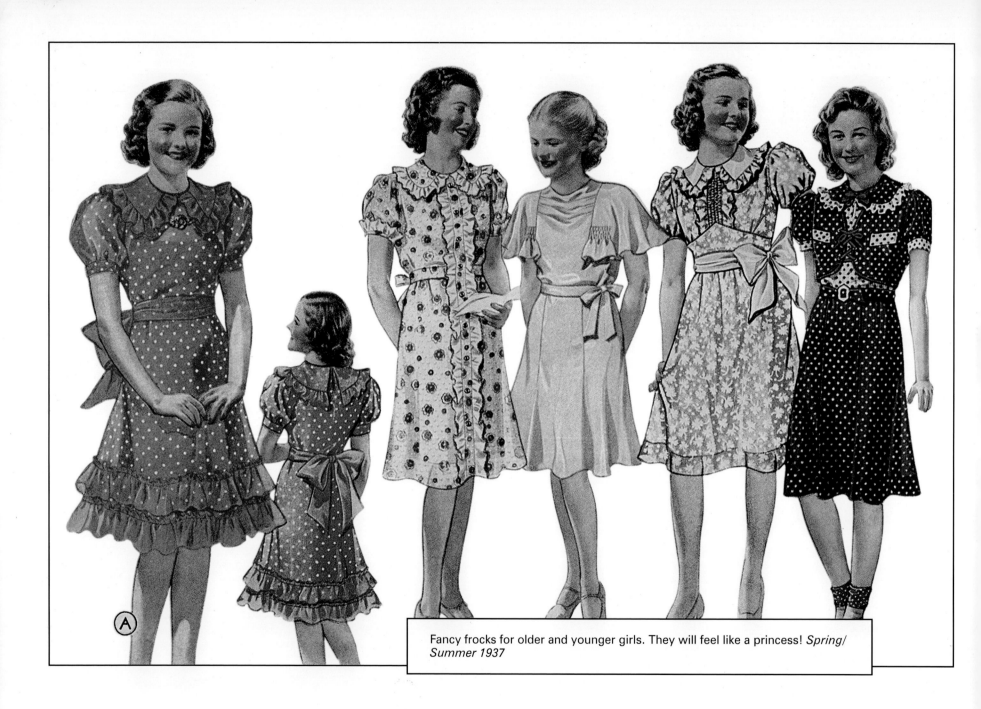

Fancy frocks for older and younger girls. They will feel like a princess! *Spring/ Summer 1937*

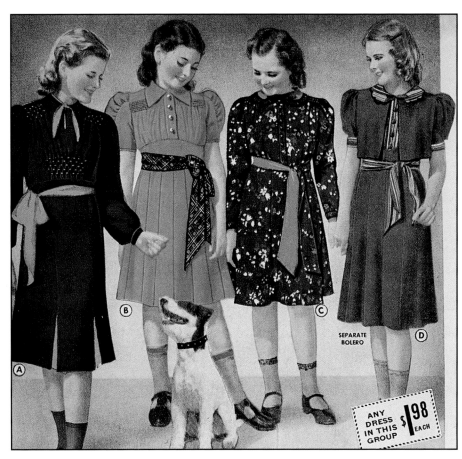

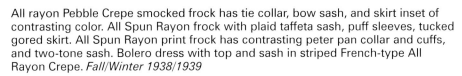

All rayon Pebble Crepe smocked frock has tie collar, bow sash, and skirt inset of contrasting color. All Spun Rayon frock with plaid taffeta sash, puff sleeves, tucked gored skirt. All Spun Rayon print frock has contrasting peter pan collar and cuffs, and two-tone sash. Bolero dress with top and sash in striped French-type All Rayon Crepe. *Fall/Winter 1938/1939*

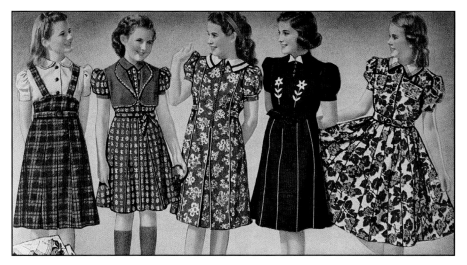

"Classmates" and "Butterfly" frocks in many styles and colors. *Fall/Winter 1938/1939*

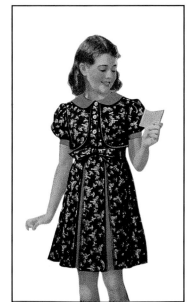

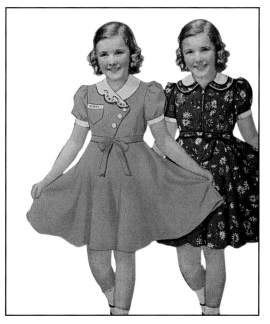

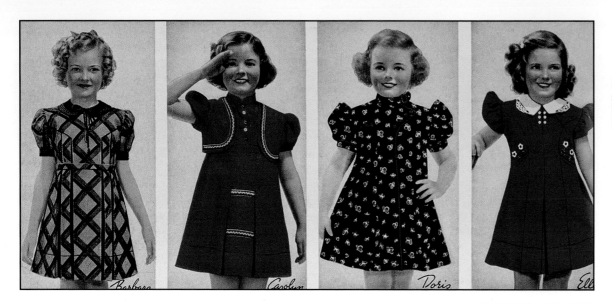

Dresses for little girls are made in exclusive styles, better fabrics, guaranteed wash fast, better dressmaking and designing, and have deep 4" hems. *Fall/Winter 1937-1938*

Bolero frock in two-tone combination. Multi-Color Dot pattern with embroidered lawn collar. "Searspride" Sailor in percale with white braid trim on sleeves and collar. "Searspride" princess buttons down the front, has tie-back sash, and piping down the front, on collar, and pockets. *Fall/ Winter 1937-1938*

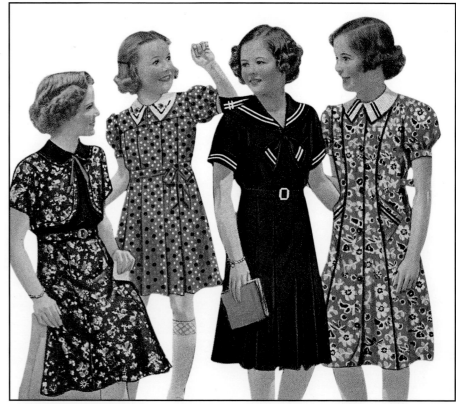

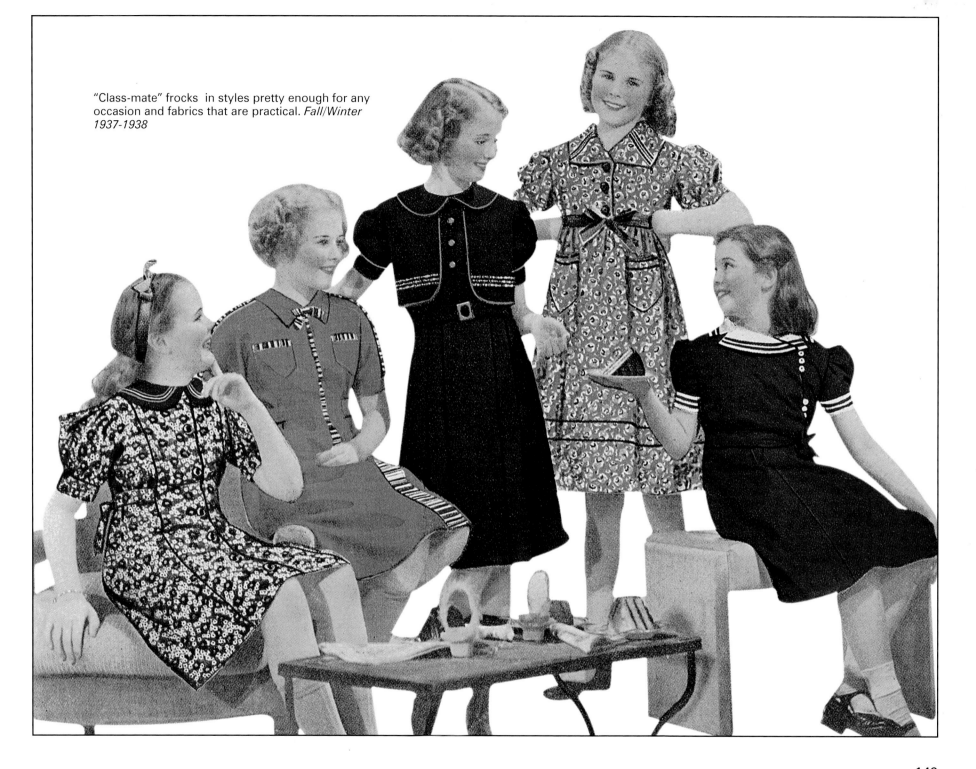

"Class-mate" frocks in styles pretty enough for any occasion and fabrics that are practical. *Fall/Winter 1937-1938*

Coats

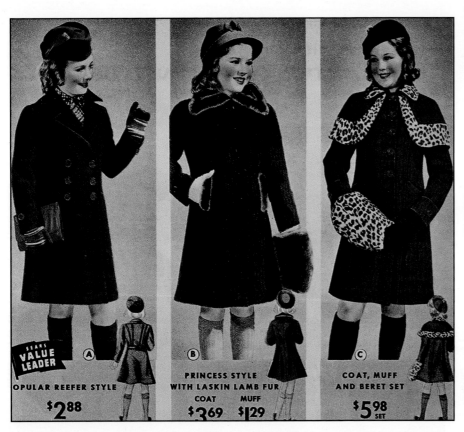

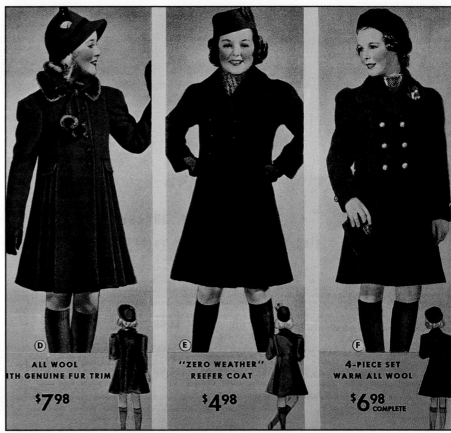

Reefer style half wool coat. Laskin Lamb fur trimmed Princess model in half wool. Coat, beret, and muff in half wool. *Fall/Winter 1938/1939*

"Classmates" coats in all wool Princess trimmed with genuine Coney fur. Double-breasted Coachman style is extra heavy soft fleece. 4-piece all wool Princess set has matching purse, beret, and bright plaid scarf. *Fall/Winter 1938/1939*

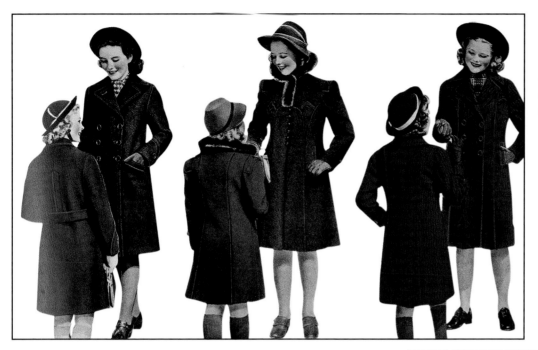

"Classmates" coats in styles and sizes for little girls to young teens. *Fall/Winter 1938/1939*

Classmates coats in smart styles, rich fabrics, and fine tailoring. *Fall/Winter 1937-1938*

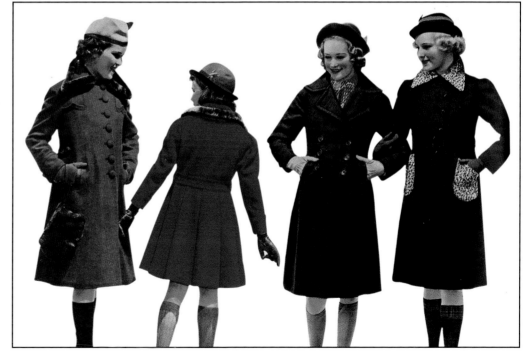

Sportswear

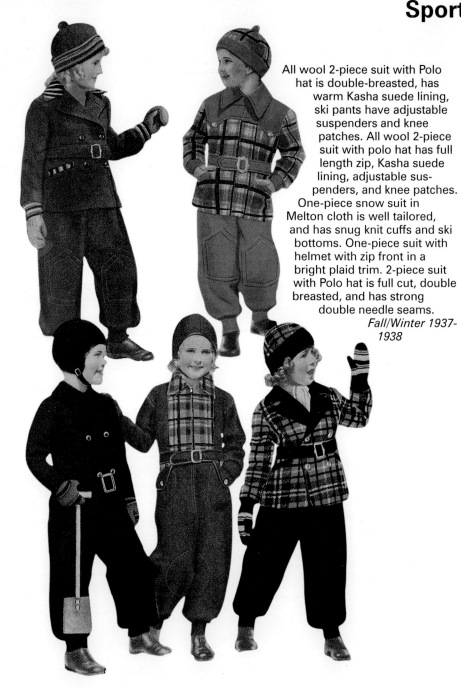

All wool 2-piece suit with Polo hat is double-breasted, has warm Kasha suede lining, ski pants have adjustable suspenders and knee patches. All wool 2-piece suit with polo hat has full length zip, Kasha suede lining, adjustable suspenders, and knee patches. One-piece snow suit in Melton cloth is well tailored, and has snug knit cuffs and ski bottoms. One-piece suit with helmet with zip front in a bright plaid trim. 2-piece suit with Polo hat is full cut, double breasted, and has strong double needle seams. *Fall/Winter 1937-1938*

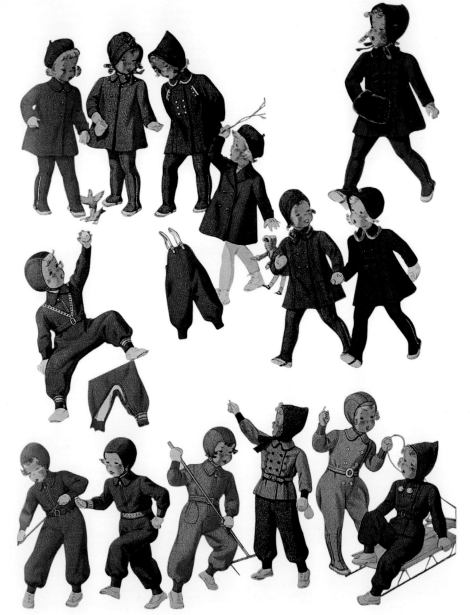

Assorted styles and colors of children's coat sets to keep them warm for outdoor fun and exercise. *Fall/Winter 1939-1940*

Undergarments

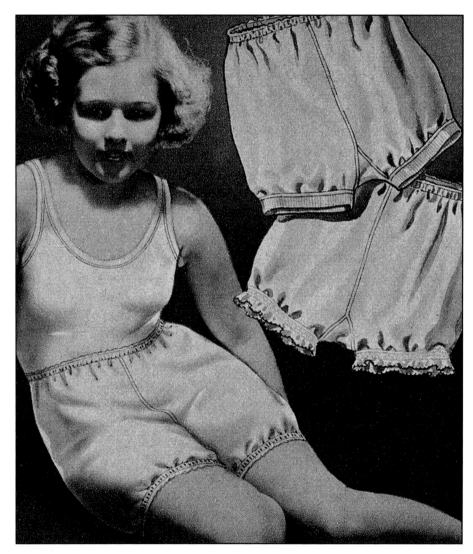

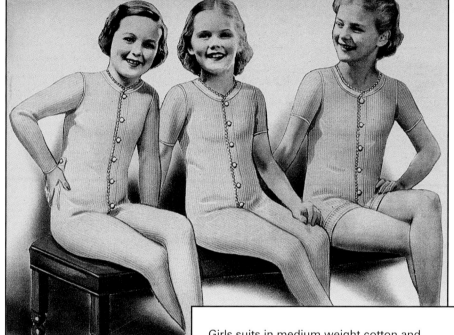

Girls suits in medium weight cotton and lightly fleeced for extra warmth. Short leg style elastic ribbed knit cotton suits. 10% wool rayon striped suits mixed with selected cotton has dainty picot edging and rayon trim on the Dutch neck. Fleeced cotton suit is the warmest suit you can buy. *Fall/Winter 1937-1938*

Girls' knit rayon vests, bloomers, and panties. *Fall/Winter 1937-1938*

Boys

Suits

Single and Double breasted suits of overplaid cassimere, wool, balance cotton and rayon. Both suits have pleated sports back with half belt jackets, cotton broadcloth button-on shirts, and cuff bottom longies. *Fall/Winter 1938/ 1939*

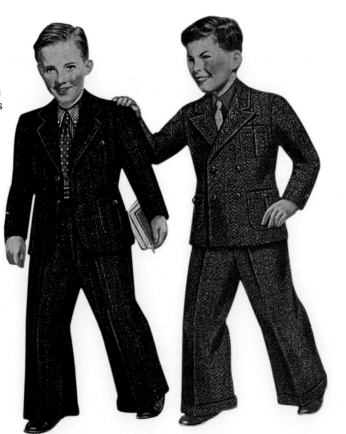

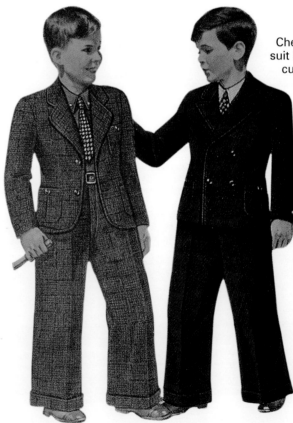

Checked pattern cassimere suit has Rugby style coat and cuff bottom longies. Navy Blue cheviot double-breasted suit has sport back coat and cuff bottom longies. *Fall/ Winter 1937-1938*

Casual Wear

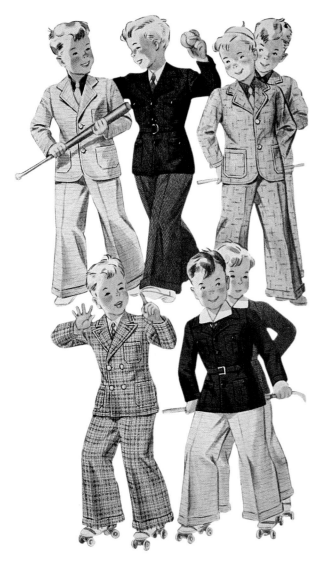

5-piece suits for boys includes coat (single or double breasted), longies, belt and tie. For less formal occasions the "Bush" suit includes coat, longies, and belt. *Spring/Summer 1939*

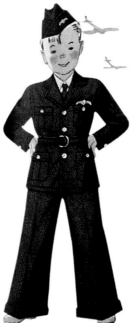

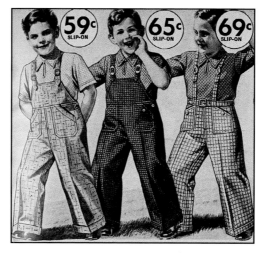

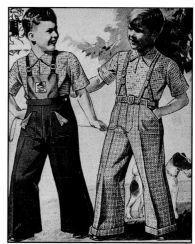

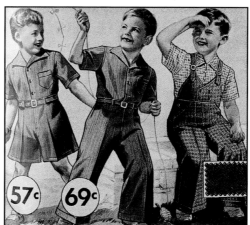

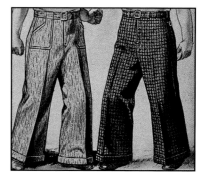

Built stronger to wear longer, these bibs, longies, slacks, camp suits, and suspenders can keep up with your boys! *Spring/Summer 1937*

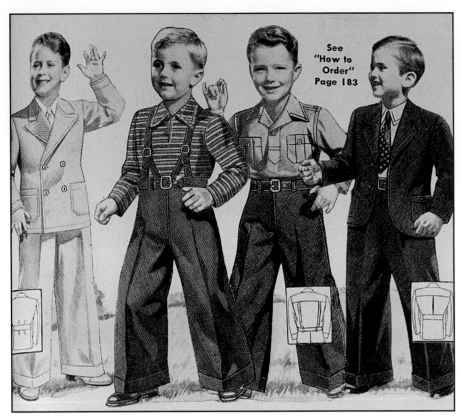

Gabardine suit in all white for those special occasions. Suspender longie suit is a favorite for boys. Three-piece suit includes shirt, longies, and belt. Five-piece suit in Navy Blue includes coat, longies with self belt, shirt and tie. *Spring/Summer 1938*

A large selection of boys clothing for the summer of 1938. *Spring/Summer 1938*

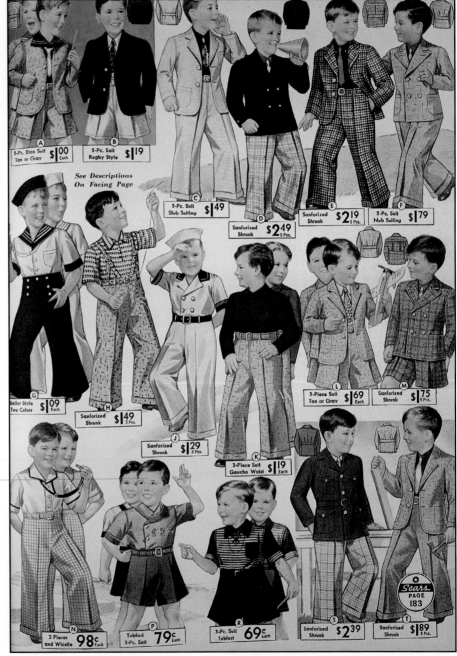

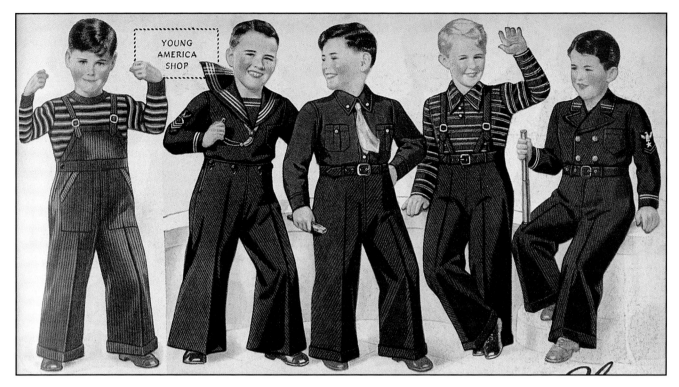

Bib outfit of brown heavy corduroy and bright striped cotton jersey. Sailor suit has twill blouse, button on longies, with cord and whistle. Sports back suit with cheviot longies, cotton broadcloth button on shirt, with self belt and tie. Suspender suit in navy blue cotton twill with blue striped cotton jersey. Admiral Jr. blue cotton twill suit has double-breasted button on shirt. *Fall/Winter 1938/1939*

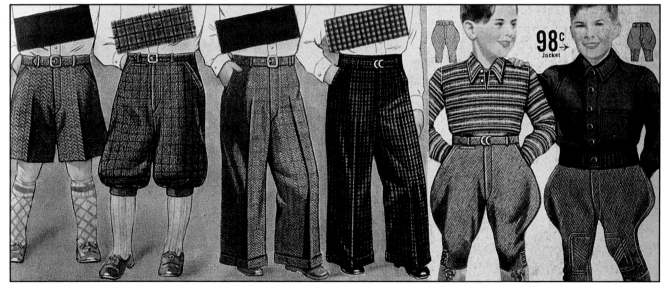

Cheviot or Cassimere lined shorts with self belt and 3 pockets. Check pattern lined knickers with self belt buckle. Tailored longies has fly front with 3 pockets. Thickset corduroy slacks hard front pleats and cuff bottoms. Cotton Whipcord Breeches and blouses make a fine school outfit. Jacket and breeches are great for winter fun. *Fall/Winter 1938/1939*

Action Playwear

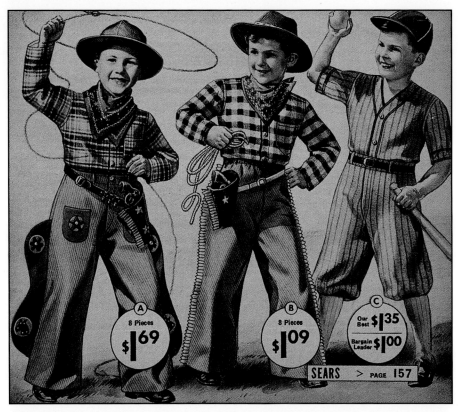

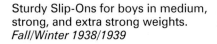

Texas Ranger and Rough Rider outfits are an 8-piece set. Play Ball outfit is a 4-piece set. Everything your little cowboy or ballplayer needs to have fun. *Spring/Summer 1937*

Sturdy Slip-Ons for boys in medium, strong, and extra strong weights. *Fall/Winter 1938/1939*

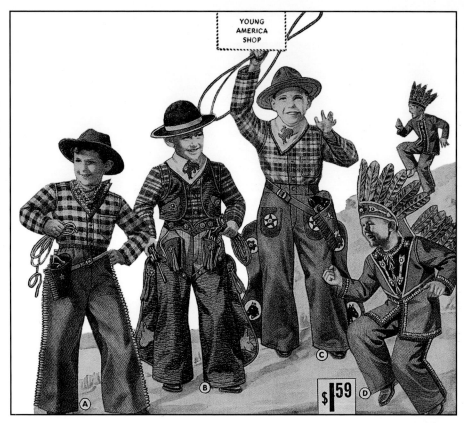

Wild West Togs for your active boys in Rough Rider, Two-Gun Pete, Bronco Buster, and Heap Big Injun. *Fall/Winter 1938/1939*

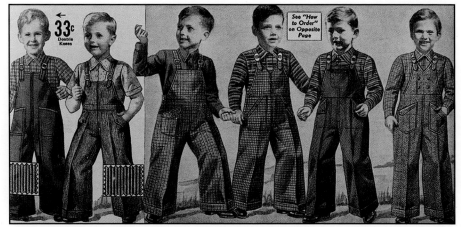

Underwear

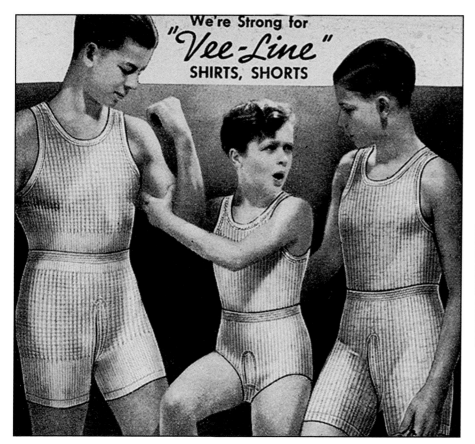

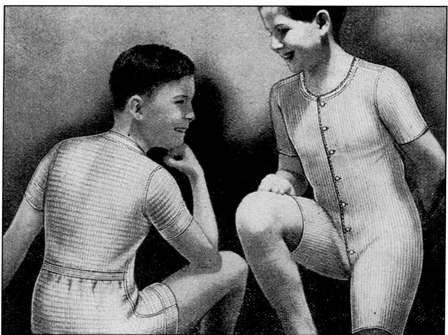

Boys underwear in medium and light weights. *Fall/Winter 1937-1938*

Family Swimwear

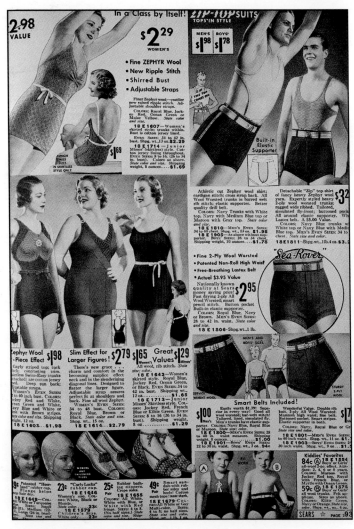

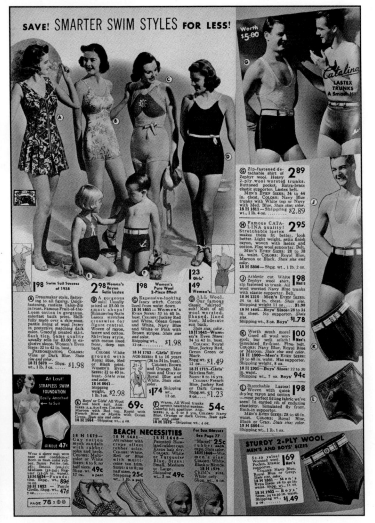

Head to the beach with swimming suits and gear for the whole family. *Spring/Summer 1937*

All the necessities your family needs for a trip to the beach in the latest styles and colors. *Spring/Summer 1938*